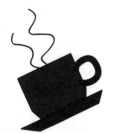

Special Diets for Special Kids Two

New! More Great Tasting Recipes & Tips for
Implementing Special Diets to Aid in the Treatment of
Autism and Related Developmental Disorders

by Lisa Lewis, Ph.D.

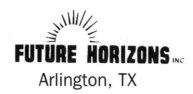

FUTURE HORIZONS INC
Arlington, TX

All marketing and publishing rights

guaranteed to and reserved by

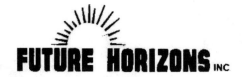

FUTURE HORIZONS INC.

Future Horizons
721 W. Abram Street
Arlington, TX 76013

800-489-0727; 817-277-0727
817-277-2270 Fax

Website: www.FutureHorizons-autism.com
E-mail: info@FutureHorizons-autism.com

ISBN# 1-885477-81-3

Table of Contents

Preface

In the four years since **Special Diets for Special Kids** was published, I have met and corresponded with thousands of parents who use dietary intervention to help their autistic spectrum children. In that time, the question I am most often asked is, "When are you publishing more recipes?"

At long last, here is the second volume of **Special Diets!**

There are now so many people following a gluten and casein free diet that I questioned whether this book was even necessary. After all, fifteen minutes on the Internet is likely to yield more recipes than are gathered here. Others have assured me, however, that they do want my "take" on recipes, and that it would be useful to have some of the best ones all in one place. And so a sequel was born.

This book is not intended to replace the first, and if you have not read **Special Diets for Special Kids** you should—it is in the first volume that I have gathered the research underlying the diet and explained it fully. This book covers the same material in only a cursory way. I have also included some material that was not available when the first volume was published.

The second question I am most often asked is, "How is Sam doing—has he recovered?" That question is harder to answer because, like most families, we have had many ups and downs.

As I write, Sam is thirteen years old. As everyone knows, adolescence is never an easy time and though we are just at the start of the hormonal roller coaster, I expect we are in for a "thrilling" ride. Sam has not recovered but continues to do well in many respects. He is extremely verbal, and is fully capable of conversation (though typically he prefers his own subjects to those of others). He attended a regular elementary school (with a personal aide and a great deal of support) for four years, and last year attended sixth grade at a private school for people with various disabilities.

Moving Sam to a private, "special" placement was a difficult decision for us. We felt that he had gained much by being with typical peers, but as we entered those difficult middle school grades, we did not believe he could fit in enough to have friends. While our local schools met his academic needs very well, as he gets older, we believe he needs an environment that can offer life skills training as well as academics.

Sam still struggles with self-control and it is his tendency to explode that prevents him from fulfilling his promise. Sam understands the importance of self-control and is always contrite after a tantrum. It is heartbreaking when he cries and says, "It was all my fault" after a tantrum is over. Still, understanding the need for calm and being able to maintain it are two different things. For that reason, we continue to use medication and it helps quite a bit.

For many children, diet alone can control outbursts. But for Sam it has never been enough. We have also found, only recently, that a supplement called Colostrum Gold has helped to stabilize Sam's moods. This supplement is usually given to help boost the immune system and it reputedly helps to heal leaky guts. It is also credited as an important tool in the anti-yeast arsenal. No one really understands why this natural supplement would help with Sam's mood stabilization, but that is our experience.

Despite behavioral challenges, Sam continues to grow and improve and very often makes us proud.

Last year, capitalizing on Sam's love of books and libraries, my husband Serge met with our local librarians to discuss a volunteer job for Sam. For the past ten months, Sam has gone "to work" one evening a week, reporting to a librarian who agreed to supervise him. He finds mis-shelved books, sorts magazines (by date and alphabetically) and does other useful tasks assigned to him. For now at least, Sam is happy with his "pay" —checking out books about U.S. states or foreign countries.

In **Special Diets for Special Kids**, I ended Chapter 1 with the questions:

Will Sam become an independent adult?

Will he get through school? Hold down a job?

Will he have real friends who share his interests?

How will the story end?

When I wrote these questions I did not know the answers, and I still do not. We keep on trying, and working towards those goals. We may not make it, but if we do not try we'll never know.

I do know that Sam always surprises us with what he can do, and this makes all our efforts worthwhile.

Lisa Lewis

July 2001

Foreword

All parents are busy. But parents of children with autism and other disabilities take "busy" to new heights. Dietary intervention has helped so many kids with autism that it is necessary to try the diet, and to do it right. But, oh, man, our brains are *full*. I mean, *crammed* with information. I don't have to tell you that the stress associated with raising autistic children makes learning new things even harder. When our lives are already pushed to the limit, how can we possibly begin to cook and prepare food in an entirely different manner than we've ever done before?

I'll let you in on a little secret. When interventions make a difference, your efforts will be paid back a hundred times over. If your child is a "diet responder," every new glimmer of understanding, every bit of imaginative play, every new word learned will serve to reward, to motivate, and to inspire you.

The news gets even better—someone has already cleared the path!

The "grunt" work has been done—by a remarkable mom with a true knack for cooking and a real way with words. Lisa's books are not only helpful, they're fun and easy to read.

Special Diets for Special Kids was a landmark book. In a world where so little was known about dietary intervention for autism, it gave parents the *reasons* for the diet, the *directions* for the diet, and the *recipes* we needed to keep our kids from starving. I estimate that, back in 1995, I went more than $25,000 into debt to get my hands on the very information in Lisa Lewis' first book. I envy those of you who are just getting started and have her books at your fingertips, but I'm so glad to know that your way will be easier than mine. The faster you can get hold of this information, the better you can help your children.

Despite my initial fumbling and bumbling, my son was one of the lucky ones who began early and responded dramatically to the removal of gluten and casein. He left the autistic spectrum years ago, but the diet is still a fact of life for him. I am teaching him to cook, and we use a very fine "textbook."

Thanks to Lisa, he won't spend his life glumly eating rice and baked potatoes. He'll eat pancakes, omelettes, sandwiches, tortillas, shepherd's pies, vegetables, snacks, pastries, cookies, and baked goods that will make him the envy of his friends (and probably the healthiest of his peers).

Aside from a few delicious meals that Lisa let us guinea pig, the content of this book is new to me—I have been eagerly awaiting its debut as much as every other GF/CF family. Even though I am an "old pro" at the diet, I don't have time to search out, test, or create many new recipes. Just like her many other fans, I count on Lisa for that.

Karyn Seroussi, Author

Unraveling the Mystery of Autism and PDD

June, 2001

Caution

Lately, ground meat has been found to occasionally be contaminated with *Escherichia coli* bacteria, more commonly known as *E. coli*. These bacteria are potentially deadly, especially for young children, the elderly, and those with weak or compromised immune systems.

All ground meat, therefore, should be cooked until thoroughly done—155 degrees Fahrenheit. Cooking the meat to this temperature will ensure that all bacteria are dead, and that your family is safe.

If you prefer ground meat that is not well-done, you can lessen the risk by ensuring that you buy only the very best ground meat, or that you buy the whole cuts and grind them yourself.

Whatever you do, use hot, soapy water to wash your hands, any utensils you might have used, and any contaminated surfaces.

Caution

Raw eggs occasionally contain *Salmonella enteritidis,* a bacterium which can cause illness and even death. Be sure to handle raw eggs carefully, especially when cooking for those with compromised or weak immune systems.

Buy fresh eggs and keep them refrigerated. If an egg looks or smells doubtful, don't use it. Saving the cost of one egg isn't worth the possible illness that egg could cause.

Be sure to cook each egg to an internal temperature of 140 degrees Fahrenheit. This will kill any bacteria in the egg. At this temperature whites will be firm and opaquely white, and yolks will be solid all the way through.

After handling raw eggs, be sure to use hot, soapy water to wash your hands, utensils, and any surfaces with which the raw eggs may have come in contact. This will prevent cross-contamination of other foods and cooking utensils.

While only about one in 10,000 eggs is contaminated with *S. enteritidis,* it's just not worth the risk to handle any raw egg carelessly.

Chapter 1
Introduction

(Q&A)

There is little question that the rate of autism has been climbing, although the reasons behind the increase are the subject of vigorous debate. Some still try to argue that better reporting and diagnosis explains the increase, but as the numbers continue to rise the silliness of this explanation becomes apparent. Just how hard is it to diagnose a child on the autistic spectrum? Have parents and doctors truly been so clueless that they were missing these kids? To anyone who has ever lived with an autistic spectrum disability child, this is ridiculous.

What is clear is this—the number of children who were "born autistic" (i.e., they were different from birth or shortly thereafter) does not appear to have changed. When experts say that autism is "rare," they are probably right, if they are referring only to this sub-group of individuals.

What seems to be increasing at an alarming pace is the number of children with a "regressive" form of the disorder. These children develop normally for up to two years, and then development either stops or they lose skills already acquired. For these children, autism is probably not due to a defect in brain development, but is more likely to be a brain dysfunction that is secondary to extraneous factors, such as metabolic or immune dysfunctions, infections or toxins.

For many of these children, the regression began nearly concurrently with routine childhood immunizations. So far, much money and energy have been expended proving that there is no causal connection between the vaccinations and autism; parents are demanding that we spend at least as much on finding out if the

1

association is causal and if so, for which children. No one argues that vaccinations are an important component of public health. However, if immunizations, or some component of them, are found to be harmful for some children, we must try to determine who should avoid them.

If we focus on the biological basis of autistic spectrum disorders, a pattern emerges:

- A child may be genetically predisposed to improper immune response.

- Some "load" triggers abnormal immune response. This load may be vaccines, or some component of vaccines.

- The child is frequently ill due to decreased immunity.

- Antibiotics are given (though infections are often viral).

- "Good" gut flora are wiped out; *Candida* (yeast) overgrowth causes gut damage.

- Mercury in vaccines may inhibit enzymes needed to break down peptides.

- An inability to process certain proteins such as gluten and casein develops, perhaps because of enzyme deficiency.

- Improperly digested peptides escape the damaged gut into the bloodstream.

- Opioid peptides mimic neurotransmitters and scramble signals.

Why Dietary Intervention for Autism?

The idea of dietary intervention has its origins in 1980, when scientist Jaak Panksepp observed that autistic children had many traits in common with people addicted to opioid drugs. Addicts are often "in their own world," and frequently exhibit stereotypic behaviors (e.g., rocking). Generally, opiate addicts are insensitive to pain and have serious gastrointestinal problems. Panksepp proposed that autistic children might have elevated levels of naturally occurring opioids in their central nervous systems.

These observations led to research in Norway, Great Britain and the United States. In all locations, abnormal peptides were found in the urine of autistic children. These findings ultimately resulted in the postulation of what is now called the "opioid excess theory" of autism. [For more information please refer to **Special Diets for Special Kids** (1998. Future Horizons: Arlington, Texas)]. Briefly, this hypothesis suggests that autism and its associated symptoms result from the incomplete breakdown of peptides derived from foods that contain gluten and casein, and also to excessive absorption of these peptides (due to a "leaky gut"). According to the theory's proponents, the presence of these peptides causes disruption to biochemical and neuroregulatory processes in the brain.

Recent research at Johnson & Johnson has confirmed the presence of these substances in the urine of autistic subjects. Perhaps more significant, another urinary compound was found and identified in autistic subjects. Known as *dermorphin*, this highly hallucinogenic substance was not found in the urine of any non-autistic person.

How on earth did this get into the urine of autistic children? One theory is that it is a fungal metabolite—in other words, there is a fungal infection and dermorphin is the byproduct of the metabolism of that organism. This may be why some children with autism respond well to an anti-yeast diet and treatment with anti-fungal medications.

We hope that soon someone will positively identify the enzyme or enzymes which are inactive or insufficiently active to metabolize these common dietary proteins. For now, however, all these researchers have one thing in common:

All recommend that gluten and casein be removed from the diet of autistic spectrum children.

Until researchers discover why these proteins are not broken down, removal of the proteins from the diet remains the only way to prevent further damage. Some children who were diagnosed with autism and began the diet before the age of two have lost their labels and no longer need medical or special education services. For children who started the diet at a later age, this level of recovery may be out of reach. Even so, thousands of parents around the world will attest to the dramatic improvement that can be achieved by implementing a GF/CF dietary program.

So, has the "opioid excess" theory been proven? No, if by proof you mean double-blind, placebo-controlled studies. As of this writing several researchers are designing such studies and seeking funding. We do have some excellent data from so-called "open studies" done in the United States and Europe, and overwhelming anecdotal evidence from this country and abroad. Most theories are investigated because of the existence of anecdotal evidence, so don't be discouraged by doctors who dismiss it on the grounds that all data are "only anecdotal."

The opiate theory "explains" the symptoms, and at least six independent labs have found abnormal peptides in the urine of ASD children—peptides which are not found in the urine of normal controls. Clearly something is putting them there. Since removal of foods containing gluten and casein leads to widespread improvement, it makes sense to assume that the foods are the source. Removing the foods is the next logical step.

Recently, I have received many letters from parents questioning the safety of soy protein for children on the gluten-free/casein-free (GF/CF) diet. Dr. William Shaw from the Great Plains Lab in Overton, Kansas, has concerns about soy because of some cross-reactivity in his test for casomorphin. While we cannot yet say for sure whether or not soy can turn into the same kind of mischievous peptides we believe to come from dairy and gluten, we do know that soy protein is structurally similar to dairy protein, and soy allergy is common in babies and children with milk allergy. In fact, a recent abstract from the Committee on Nutrition at the American Academy of Pediatrics (AAP) states:

> **Severe gastrointestinal reactions to soy protein formula have been described for greater than 30 years, and encompass the full gamut of disease seen with cow milk protein in infancy: enteropathy, enterocolitis, and proctitis. Small-bowel injury, a reversible celiac-like villus injury that produces an enteropathy with malabsorption, hypoalbuminemia, and failure to thrive, has been documented in at least four studies. To date, those afflicted have responded to the elimination of soy protein-based formulas and are no longer sensitive by 5 years of age.**
>
> **Severe enterocolitis manifested by bloody diarrhea, ulcerations, and histologic features of acute and chronic inflammatory bowel disease also has been well described in infants receiving soy protein-based formulas. They respond quickly to elimination of the soy formula and introduction of a hydrolyzed protein formula. Their degree of sensitivity to**

soy protein during the first few years of age can remain dramatic; thus, casual use of soy-based formula is to be avoided. Most children, *but not all,* can resume soy protein consumption safely after 5 years of age.

In addition, up to 60% of infants with cow milk protein-induced enterocolitis also will be equally sensitive to soy protein. It is theorized that the intestinal mucosa damaged by cow milk allows increased uptake and, therefore, increased immunologic response to the subsequent antigen soy. Eosinophilic proctocolitis, a more benign variant of enterocolitis, also has been reported in infants receiving soy protein-based formula.

These dietary protein-induced syndromes of enteropathy and enterocolitis, although clearly immunologic in origin, are not immunoglobulin E-mediated, reflecting instead an age-dependent transient soy protein hypersensitivity. Because of the reported high frequency of infants sensitive to both cow milk and soy antigens, soy protein-based formulas are not indicated in the management of documented cow milk protein-induced enteropathy or enterocolitis."

In other, simpler words, if milk allergy is a problem, soy allergy is likely to be a problem too. And just as milk intolerance can lead to GI problems, but is often outgrown after five years of strict avoidance, the same may be true of soy intolerance. However, the question still remains: can soy peptides lead to autistic behaviors?

According to Dr. Shaw, an extremely high percentage of the autistic children he tests for food allergies show reactivity to soy as well as milk. Soy is known to be one of the most allergenic foods, and although it is a legume, its protein is structurally similar to that of milk. He has also heard from a few parents that soy seems to affect behavior. Is this because of allergy and discomfort? Or is it due to the uptake of "tofumorphin?"

So, what should you do about soy? Removing soy certainly limits the diet even further, but it seems prudent to remove it temporarily to see if there is further improvement. At the Autism Network for Dietary Intervention (ANDI), Karyn Seroussi and I are now suggesting that all kids on the GF/CF diet should have a 2-3 week no-soy trial. You can then try rotating it back in, with a "soy day" every fourth day. Keep a behavior diary for a few weeks. On or after a soy day, if there are no ill effects on conduct, activity level, discomfort, sleep, skin, or bowels, you should be able to put soy back in the diet on a regular basis. Dr. Shaw agrees that this is a reasonable approach, and indicates that he will have more information on this subject as he completes further studies in his lab.

Dr. Ted Kniker of the San Antonio Autistic Treatment Center in Texas found that, out of 28 children and adults with autism, five showed improvements in their symptoms after elimination of dairy products and wheat glutens from their diets. In the second part of the study, Kniker eliminated additional foods, including buckwheat, tomatoes, soy, pork and grapes.

Symptoms changed dramatically in 39.3% of patients during the second phase of the 3-month intervention period," he said. Eight out of 28 patients showed clear improvements, as measured by a variety of quantitative scoring methods, including the Autistic Treatment Evaluation Checklist. Of course, by eliminating more than one food at a time, this study makes it impossible to know if *all* these foods needed to be eliminated. Further research is needed and is planned.

Some of the recipes in this book do include soy, though there are nearly always alternatives listed. I did try a soy-free period for our son and saw no negative reaction when soy was added back to his diet. Further, he did not give a positive result on any of the laboratory tests to casomorphin after being dairy free for many years (despite a high intake of soy).

If your child can tolerate soy, it is a good way to add protein and variety to the diet. However, if soy is a no-no, you will be glad you have eliminated it from the diet. So please, take the time to do a no-soy trial before using it freely in your child's diet.

Like cow's milk, soy is becoming a controversial food. It is an excellent cash crop and a great source of protein (especially for vegetarians), but there are several cautionary tales about soy isoflavones. Many of these strike me as anti-soy propaganda, but there's just as much propaganda hailing soy as an important food. Because it is too soon to give a definitive answer as to whether or not you should use soy, I encourage you to research the topic yourself; you can start with a visit to the website: **http://www.fda.gov/fdac/features/2000/300_soy.html**

For years autism has been likened to a puzzle; the ASA logo incorporates this theme, as do the "autism ribbons" available at conferences around the world. This diet is clearly one piece to that puzzle. For a large number of autistic spectrum children, it seems to be the most critical piece. For others it will help, but less dramatically. For a smaller number it does not seem to be a significant piece of the puzzle.

Even for the sub-group of children greatly helped by dietary intervention, it is important to try to balance the entire system. ASD kids are notorious for their deficiencies in various minerals and amino acids. They eat terrible diets and their leaky guts don't allow for good absorption of nutrients anyway. It is critically important that we get them into the best nutritional state we can; if we do this we are more likely to see good results from diet or whatever "puzzle piece" is needed for a particular child.

Since forming the ANDI with Karyn Seroussi, we have heard from over ten thousand parents. We know that this group is self-selecting—we are less likely to hear from parents of children who did not benefit from the diet. What is clear, however, is that the children with the regressive type of autism seem to be the ones most likely to respond to dietary intervention. If started early enough, some recover. Others improve significantly. The letter on page 10 is typical of those we receive.

November 20, 2000

Dear Lisa:

Our son was diagnosed as autistic 3 weeks ago, and we have had him on the GF/CF diet for 10 days. Wow!

The changes we have seen since beginning the diet include:

SLEEP: Instead of waking 1-3 times per night, he has slept through EVERY night!

BOWEL MOVEMENTS: We were using apricot nectar, and occasional suppositories to soften his stool.   He has had "normal looking baby poop" since the diet.

SPEECH: Over the last 3-4 months all language was lost.   Since the diet, speech has returned and new words have been added.   He is even putting two words together!

EYE CONTACT: Eye contact has improved; now we can get his attention.

INCREASED APPETITE: He is eating more foods!

TANTRUMS: Have gone from 10 a day to 3 a week!

FOCUS: He has come out of the fog he was in!

You have given us hope that our son will have a good and productive life,

THANK YOU!!

[Name withheld]

Whenever I speak to parents, whether they are diet "newbies" or old hands, the same questions always arise. I am certain that readers of this book will have some of the same questions (particularly if they ignored the advice to read **Special Diets for Special Kids** first.) I hope that by answering some of these questions "up front," you will be encouraged either to start this dietary intervention, or to stick with it.

Frequently Asked Questions

Will this diet help with other disorders?

Many times parents choose to put the whole family on the diet, either for the convenience of preparing only one meal, or because the child is sneaking gluten- and casein-containing foods. Often, parents report that their child's ADHD siblings improved dramatically, or that seizures decreased (or stopped), or even that their own migraines have disappeared. Shattock reports (in a personal communication) that several people with obsessive-compulsive disorder have improved dramatically when on the GF/CF diet.[1] Some parents who have used the Feingold Diet (see **http://www.feingold.org** for more information) find that combining this additive-free diet with a gluten and casein free diet is very beneficial. Many siblings who have never been diagnosed with a disorder seem to do well on the diet too. Remember, autism is a spectrum disorder; even children on the higher functioning end report good results.

---

[1] To read about research that has been done in Europe, be sure to visit Paul Shattock's website at **http://osiris.sunderland.ac.uk/autism/treat.html.**

How long must we do this diet? Is it life-long?

Beware of anyone who gives you a time frame for the diet; the fact is, we simply do not know if diet-responders can ever safely return to a "normal" diet. What we do know is this: most children seem to have dramatic reactions to dietary infractions, but only for a limited time. That period may be months or even a few years. At some point, however, a mistake or intentional infraction ceases to cause dramatic effects. Why? We don't know for sure, but it is probably due to the fact that a previously leaky gut has healed. We must assume that the underlying metabolic problem remains unchanged and the peptides are still not being fully digested. However, if the gut has healed the peptides won't get through to cause noticeable reactions.

So why not give up the diet at this point? In all likelihood a few months of eating the foods will cause damage to the gut and start the cycle all over again. I have heard from many parents who made this mistake. They stopped the diet and all was well for a time, but then the child began to deteriorate. For a few, the regression was severe and long lasting. For the time being, the wisest course is to continue the diet.

There are, unfortunately, a few companies which are trying to persuade parents that their children can go off the diet, as long as they also consume particular digestive enzymes (which of course they sell at premium prices). They encourage parents to "take the challenge" and give their children the forbidden foods along with a sample of their enzymes. Of course, if the child has been on the diet for quite a while, there is no reaction. The parents are often hoodwinked into believing that the enzymes caused this wondrous event.

Digestive enzymes can be a terrific adjunct to the diet, and are especially helpful when there has been an infraction, or if you simply are not sure about the safety of a particular food. I recommend EnZymAid (Kirkman Laboratories) and Seren-Aid (Klaire Labs). However, keep in mind that even the developers of these enzymes do not recommend that they be used instead of the diet.

We would all like a magic pill that would allow us to feed our kids like everyone else, but so far, it does not exist. Remember the old saw "if it sounds too good to be true, it probably is." And remember, "everyone else" feeds his or her kids a lot more junk than you do!

How long will it be until I see results?

That is a hard question to answer because it depends on several factors. In general, younger children respond more quickly. Typically a negative response (withdrawal) is seen within a week, followed by a positive response in 3-5 weeks. Older children and adults generally take longer to show results. It also depends on how much gluten and casein was in the diet, and on the condition of the gut.

Should I make my kids go "cold turkey?"

This is an apt term, considering how like a drug addiction these foods are to some kids. For children younger than five, a gradual removal of the foods is probably better. It is easier to remove dairy, and I usually suggest removing it over the course of a week to ten days (replaced by appropriate calcium enriched, casein free drinks). The gluten should follow. Over all, complete removal of the foods should not take more than 4-6 weeks. Older children can go cold turkey, but it is stressful and if possible should be avoided.

I have heard that I should remove corn too—is this true?

There is no question that some children must be off other foods in addition to gluten and casein. For some, the reaction to corn (or soy, or tomatoes, or eggs etc.) is even more profound than the reaction to gluten or casein. However, it may simply be a case of a food allergy or some other kind of intolerance. For some, soy and corn seem to cause no problem whatsoever.

If a child shows improvement when gluten and casein are removed but then deteriorates, you should suspect another food (or foods) of causing a problem. Once gluten and casein have been removed, soy and corn often begin to occupy a much more prominent place in the diet. These foods were probably always problematic, but because most of the diet consisted of wheat and dairy foods the parents did not notice.

If you suspect that either corn or another food may be causing problems, remove it completely for at least ten days. Then, put the food back into the diet for one day only, serving some at every meal. Watch the child carefully for at least three days. If there is no change when your child eats the food, you can assume it is safe. If you are not sure, repeat the test. Obviously, if there is a clear reaction the food should be kept completely out of the diet. Do the same test with any other food you believe to be suspect.

It is critical that you test one food at a time, however, or you will not be sure which food is causing your child's reaction. Keep a food diary, detailing everything that your child eats and his or her reaction to it. By following a diary over three or more days, you may be able to discern patterns that were otherwise not apparent. Many parents have pinned down food sensitivities this way. Also, beware of artificial colors and flavorings when you note reactions—for many children these must be removed completely.

What about yeast? Should my child be sugar free?

Many autistic spectrum kids have a problem with yeast overgrowth—this is most often the case when there has been a lot of antibiotic use, but it has also been seen in children who have rarely or never taken antibiotics! This problem is the result of a disturbed immune system, and it is relatively easy to test for. Great Smokies and Great Plains Labs both do non-invasive and inexpensive stool tests for yeast.

Should yeast overgrowth be a problem, then, yes, the child should be on a sugar-free diet until the overgrowth is cleared up. It is not as simple as removing sugar however, and you should consult a doctor and nutritionist for help. Many foods, in addition to sugar, must be avoided when treating yeast (e.g., anything fermented or potentially moldy). Often the addition of anti-fungal medication is also needed, along with over-the-counter probiotics (e.g., *lactobacillus*).

The good news is that for most, the yeast problem can eventually resolve with treatment. Unlike gluten and casein (and possibly soy or corn) the anti-yeast regimen is not indefinite. When preparing recipes in this book, you can use several substitutes that do not "feed" yeast. These include vegetable glycerin (be sure to buy 100% pure food grade), sucralose[2] (marketed as Splenda...), xylitol or stevia (xylitol and stevia are often available in health food stores, or can be purchased from mail order companies such as Miss Robens).

---

[2] Note that some doctors insist that all "artificial" sweeteners must be eliminated. Although sucralose is made from sugar, it must be classified as an artificial sweetener. Choose one of the other, non-yeast feeding sweeteners if you want to avoid all artificial additives. For many, this may be significant.

If it's not helping, when is it ok to quit?

Obviously, this diet is hard to maintain and there is little point in continuing if the diet does not help your child. Reichelt (in Norway) believes that a full year is necessary to be sure that it won't help. I think that for young children (under age five) three months is probably a good trial and that for older children, six months is long enough.

That said, however, it is critical to be sure that the diet was adhered to completely before deciding that it did not help. All too often parents insist they "did it right," only to discover that they were routinely using foods that contained gluten or casein! Don't forget the hidden glutens and caseins that can be found in nearly all pre-packaged foods.

What about school? Parties? Reinforcers?

Many parents complain about teachers, therapists or other caregivers who do not wish to comply with the dietary restrictions.

As long as the parents are willing to provide foods, there really is no reason to accept these arguments. My son's public school reserved a place in their freezer where I stored gluten-free cupcakes and cookies for those frequent classroom parties. For years, when he was doing one-on-one ABA therapy, I provided acceptable reinforcers and the therapists were happy to use them.

As for parties, try offering to bake for all the kids! At the very least, you can find out what is being served and take something similar along for your child.

If you have a small (preschool age) child, be aware that many non-food items get put into the mouth and are not gluten free. Play clay is usually made with gluten, and most glues and pastes are also forbidden. Be sure that the teachers know this. Offer to make some GF play clay if necessary (**Special Diets for Special Kids** had several recipes, and there are more to be found on the Internet). There are even recipes for bubbles available—many children pop bubbles with their mouths so this is an important consideration! And don't let your child have a turn at feeding the classroom fish—fish flakes contain gluten and are sticky enough to stay on the hands (which are invariably put in the mouth).

What if my doctor won't support this intervention, or belittles it?

The short answer: Find a new doctor!

Seriously, more and more health professionals are learning the importance of diet for many illnesses and disorders. It is important to remember, however, that education in nutrition was probably limited to a two-hour lecture at your doctor's medical school. He or she is not all that knowledgeable on this topic.

There is nothing dangerous about this diet.   In many parts of the world, millions of children grow up without eating wheat or drinking cow's milk. What is important is obtaining necessary nutrients, and you will find that a registered nutritionist will be more helpful to you than will a pediatrician. A nutritionist will help you understand what vitamins and minerals your child needs (and in what doses) and will show you alternative ways to obtain them.

What about vitamins?

Many doctors say that if a child eats a well-balanced diet, vitamin supplements are unnecessary. That may be true, but how many autistic spectrum children eat a well-balanced diet? Not many, I would guess. Even if a child does eat a variety of foods (some do, believe it or not, including my son Sam), they may not be absorbing the vitamins and minerals if their guts are leaky. It is important to work with someone knowledgeable (again, a nutritionist can help here). Many autistic spectrum children take one of the vitamin-mineral complexes that have been formulated especially for their needs. The two most popular are SupraNuThera (Kirkman) and DanPlex (**http://www.hopewellrx.com**).

Lisa Lewis'—

Rules to Live By

A little bit *will* hurt!

Food does not equal Love (it just seems like it does).

Reinforcers can be GF/CF.

Milk is the perfect food—if you happen to be a calf!

It is great to have a doctor's support, but you can do without it if you must.

Supplementation is critical.

"Miracles" take a lot of hard work!

Chapter 2
Drinks

Most American children drink too much juice! They fill up on what is essentially sugar-water, leaving less room for real food. The juices we serve may be fortified with vitamins and even calcium but there are other ways to sneak nutrition into a drink. The fact that kids on the GF/CF diet cannot have milk limits drink choices even more. My kids often choose a shake or smoothie for dessert, and there is no reason that these can't have some added nutrition too. In the recipes that follow, substituting sparkling mineral water for seltzer will add some calcium.

Please note: when milk substitute powder is called for, the recipe will specify "dry milk substitute" or "dry DariFree" (if DariFree works much better than other powders). If you prefer to use a dry soy milk substitute that will always work too. When liquid milk substitute is called for, the recipe will generally state only "milk substitute."

Purple Cow

I'm not sure how certain "floats" came to have bovine names, but the name is the only thing about this that has any relation to a dairy cow.

Ingredients

4 ounces grape juice

1 scoop lemon sorbet

4 ounces sparkling mineral water (or seltzer)

Combine everything in a glass and serve with a straw. If you prefer, combine in a blender to make a smooth cow.

Mock Orange Julius

I've never really enjoyed malls, but I do have fond memories of those delicious orange drinks. This non-dairy recipe is very similar to the drink I remember. If your child cannot tolerate citrus, try using unsweetened pineapple juice or a fruit nectar.

Ingredients

1 cup orange juice (preferably calcium fortified)

1 cup water

2 tablespoons dehydrated egg white (e.g. Just Whites)

1/4 cup sugar (or sugar substitute)

1/4 cup dry DariFree

1 heaping cup ice

1/4 teaspoon calcium powder

Blend all ingredients in a blender or food processor on high for 30 seconds, or until drink is thick and smooth.

Bananaberry Shake

A drink available at the Applebees® chain of restaurants suggested this yummy shake. If soy is tolerated, add some tofu for an extra jolt of protein. For extra calcium, add a teaspoon of calcium powder. If bananas are not tolerated, try making this shake with some fresh or canned pineapple instead.

Ingredients

2 cups crushed ice

1 ripe banana

1 cup strawberries

$^1/4$ cup DariFree or other milk substitute

$^1/4$ cup coconut milk

1 teaspoon calcium powder

Puree the fruit in your blender, and then add the other ingredients. Blend until smooth.

Fruit Smoothies

Let your imagination and your child's preferences guide your choices, then use your blender to combine any and all of the following:

Ingredients

DariFree or soy milk

Frozen fruit

Bananas

Sweetener (optional)

Ice

Calcium powder.

Adding ice will make your smoothie thick and creamy. You don't have to freeze the fruit you use, but it will make the drink thicker, too.

NY Style Egg Cream

The first night I spent as a New Yorker, I was squired around and treated to dozens of typical New York delicacies. The egg cream was one of them. As a Midwesterner I found this drink puzzling—no eggs, no cream. Every New Yorker has his or her ideas about what makes it "authentic." Because this recipe is dairy free, I don't claim it as a "real" egg cream, but I do think your child will find it a special treat.

Ingredients

1/4 cup DariFree or Soy milk

3 tablespoons chocolate syrup

6 ounces seltzer (or a sparkling mineral water that contains calcium, such as Gerolsteiner)

Combine milk substitute and chocolate syrup in the bottom of an 8-ounce glass, then fill with seltzer and stir. Serve while fizzy.

Coconut Eggnog

For many people, Christmas wouldn't be complete without eggnog. Most classic recipes call for milk and heavy cream. This version is a bit different, but rich and delicious. No reason to save it for the holidays if your family enjoys it.

Ingredients

6 eggs

1/4 cup sugar

1/4 teaspoon salt

4 cups coconut milk

1 teaspoon vanilla

Beat eggs, sugar and salt together. Stir in 2 cups coconut milk and transfer to the stove. Over low heat, warm the mixture, stirring constantly. When mixture has thickened, remove from heat. Stir in remaining coconut milk and the vanilla. Chill well before serving. Sprinkle with nutmeg if desired.

Wassail

Wassail is usually made with an apple base, but this one uses pear juice or nectar. Many of our kids don't tolerate apples, though if yours does and you prefer it, use apple cider for this wonderful drink. Best served warm, so if you're having company you might make it in a crockpot and leave it on low. This recipe makes a large batch.

Ingredients

8 cups pear juice or nectar

2 cups orange juice

Juice of two lemons

10 whole cloves

4 cinnamon sticks

Pinch of ground ginger

Pinch of nutmeg (preferably freshly grated)

Combine all ingredients in a large pot or crockpot. Bring to a boil and then lower to a slow simmer for at least two hours. If using a crockpot, let it simmer all day.

Chai

"Chai" is a word that, in much of the world, simply means tea. In the last few years, however, it has been used to describe a milky tea drink that is popular in coffee houses. It is easy to make your own, and it's a nice change of pace on a hot day. This recipe will make a powder that will keep indefinitely, and is mixed with the milk substitute of your choice.

Ingredients

2 sticks of cinnamon

1 teaspoon ginger powder

3 whole cloves

5 cardamom pods (you can find these in Indian markets)

1 peppercorn

1 allspice berry

Grind the above to a powder (a clean coffee grinder works well). Store in an airtight container.

To Make Chai (4 servings)

Heat (but don't boil) 2 cups of milk substitute.

Bring 3 cups of water to a boil with one tablespoon sugar.

Add 4 teaspoons of chai powder. Mix well and remove from heat.

Let the mixture "steep" for about ten minutes.

Pour milk substitute into four glasses and pour about 1/3 cup of the chai mixture into each cup of milk. Pour through a strainer if desired. Mix well. Chill and serve.

Frozen Fruit Cocktail

This recipe is ridiculously easy. Don't forget to add some calcium powder to bump up the nutrition. If your child tolerates soy, this is a nice way to add some protein. If soy isn't tolerated you can omit the tofu—the drink will not be as thick but it will still be good. For added protein you can add a few teaspoons of dehydrated egg or egg white.

Ingredients

8 ounces can of fruit cocktail in light syrup

1 block of silken tofu

1/3 cup cranberry juice

1/2 teaspoon calcium powder

Open fruit cocktail into a bowl with juice, and freeze. Combine frozen fruit with calcium powder, tofu and cranberry juice and blend until smooth.

Orange Freeze

Our kids can't order this at the Hard Rock Café because it would be full of milk. But if you make this at home with calcium fortified OJ, you've got a treat that contains a lot of calcium.

Ingredients

2 cups orange sorbet*

1 cup calcium fortified orange juice

1/4 cup DariFree or other milk substitute

Combine ingredients and blend until smooth.

*Note: most sorbets, while completely dairy free, contain corn. If your child cannot tolerate corn products, you will probably have to make your own. See recipe on page 193.

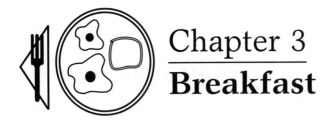

Chapter 3
Breakfast

I have always found that breakfast is the easiest meal of the day to make gluten and casein free. Because you are less dependent on yeast-risen goods, it is easier to duplicate old favorites. Products that use baking powder or soda for leavening work very well in the absence of gluten, and it is easy to "sneak" in nutrients.

Most children like breakfast foods too, which means that the table is less like a battlefield and more like a family meal. Remember, there is no law that says breakfast foods must disappear after 11 a.m. (despite what happens at fast food restaurants). If your children like and eat breakfast foods, use them all day if you want to.

Egg In The Hole

Don't ask me why, but some kids who won't eat plain fried eggs and toast will eat them if made this way. It could not be simpler.

Ingredients

2 eggs

2 slices GF bread

CF margarine

With a sharp knife, cut a small circle (approximately 2" in diameter) out of the center of each bread slice, creating a hole in the middle of each slice. Melt margarine in a fry pan over medium heat, then place bread in pan and crack egg into each hole. When almost cooked, carefully turn the egg and bread. Cook until egg is at desired degree of doneness and the bread is lightly grilled.

Easiest Pancakes

This recipe uses the Quickie Baking Mix recipe found on page 216. They are easy to make and absolutely delicious. If using DariFree, you may omit the vanilla but be sure to add it if you are using a different milk substitute. This is just one more reason to keep some of the Quickie Mix in your fridge.

Ingredients

2 cups Quickie Baking Mix

2 eggs

2 tablespoons sugar or other sweetener (optional)

1 3/4 cup (or more) DariFree or other milk substitute

1 teaspoon vanilla (optional)

Combine all ingredients. Start with a cup of the milk substitute, adding more if necessary to achieve a batter consistency (it should pour easily but should not be runny).

Heat griddle or skillet over medium-high heat or electric griddle to 375°; grease with cooking spray, vegetable oil or shortening. (Surface is ready when a few drops of water sprinkled on it dance and disappear.)

Cook until edges are dry, and then turn. Cook until golden brown and serve.

Variation: For blueberry pancakes, omit sugar and vanilla and add 1 cup fresh or frozen blueberries. Bananas or other fruits may also be used.

Gingerbread Pancakes

The International House of Pancakes® is known for its wide variety of pancakes. My favorite is their gingerbread pancakes. I don't know how IHOP makes them, but if your family likes a little spice this will make a nice change of pace for breakfast or Sunday brunch.

Ingredients

2 1/2 cups Quickie Baking Mix

1 cup (or more) DariFree (or other milk substitute)

3/4 cup apple or pear butter

2 tablespoons oil

1/2 teaspoon cinnamon

1/2 teaspoon ginger

1/2 teaspoon nutmeg

2 eggs

Combine all ingredients. Start with a cup of the milk substitute, adding more if necessary to achieve a batter consistency (it should pour easily but should not be runny).

Heat griddle or skillet over medium-high heat, or heat electric griddle to 375°; grease with cooking spray, vegetable oil or shortening (surface is ready when a few drops of water sprinkled on it dance and disappear).

Cook until edges are dry, and then turn. Cook until golden brown and serve.

Breakfast Cookies

My son loves breakfast—cereal, eggs, and pancakes—you name it. But his "typical" brother gives me fits in the morning. I can't bear to send him off to school without something nutritious, but it is always a battle. I know the same is true for many other parents, but I may have the answer for you in these breakfast cookies. These cookies pack a powerful nutrition punch. They have calcium (from the DariFree and calcium powder), protein (from the egg, nuts and bean flour), iron (from raisins), and essential fatty acids (from the flax powder). They're not terribly sweet and are easily modified for yeast-free regimens. I like this recipe so much that it has already appeared in **The ANDI News** *and in* **The Autism-Asperger Digest Magazine.** *Don't be put off by the long list of ingredients— they are easy to make.*

Ingredients

1 stick CF margarine, softened

1/3 cup pure maple syrup*

1 egg

1/2 cup orange juice*

1 1/2 teaspoons GF vanilla

1 cup GF flour blend (I like Hagman's 4 flour bean flour)

1/3 cup rice bran

1 teaspoon baking powder

1 1/2 teaspoons xanthan gum

1 teaspoon salt

1/3 cup DariFree® powder

1 cup THIN sliced poha (rice flakes, available at Indian markets or through Miss Roben's)

1/3 cup ground pecans (or other nuts, if tolerated)

1 tablespoon calcium powder (available from Kirkman Laboratories)

1 tablespoon Nutriflax powder (available in the refrigerator section of many
health food stores)

1 cup raisins* (or other dried fruit)

1/4 cup unsweetened coconut

Preheat oven to 350°.

Spray cookie sheets with vegetable oil spray.

Cream together margarine and sweetener in a large bowl. Beat in egg. Add bran,
juice, and vanilla. Add dry ingredients. Mix well. Stir in raisins and nuts and drop
on greased cookie sheet, 2 inches apart. Bake 10-12 minutes.

*If you are avoiding yeast, you can use 100 per cent pure vegetable glycerin fla-
vored with GF maple flavoring, instead of maple syrup. This very sweet liquid does
not feed yeast. Squeeze fresh orange juice immediately before making the cookies
to avoid any fermentation (often a problem with juices made from concentrate, or
that have been in the refrigerator for any period of time). Omit dried fruit.

Granola Bars I

Here's another sneaky way to get your child to eat breakfast. These also make a great after school snack. Or put them in the lunchbox on school days.

Ingredients

2 cups GF granola (see recipe on page 36)

1/2 cup GF flour blend (use a bean blend if possible for extra protein)

1/2 teaspoon baking powder

1/2 teaspoon baking soda

1 cup unsweetened applesauce*

1 teaspoon vanilla

1 teaspoon cinnamon

1 egg, beaten

1/2 cup sunflower nuts

1/2 cup coconut

1/4 cup raisins

1/4 cup dried cherries or blueberries

Heat oven to 350°. Grease 8 or 9-inch square pan.

In large bowl, combine all ingredients; mix well. Pour into prepared pan. Bake for 25 to 35 minutes or until toothpick inserted in center comes out clean. Cool. Cut into bars.

*If your child cannot eat apples, substitute with pear sauce. You can make it yourself or use baby food pears; if using baby food, be sure that there are no fillers or additives.

Granola Bars II

This recipe is chewier and much sweeter—more like a dessert than breakfast.

Ingredients

1/2 cup brown sugar

1/2 cup pure cane syrup or GF brown rice syrup

1/2 cup CF margarine, melted

1/3 cup nut butter

1 tablespoon vanilla

4 cups granola

1/2 cup coconut

1/3 cup amaranth flakes (available from Gluten Solutions)

Preheat oven to 350°.

Combine the first five ingredients and stir well. Add the granola, coconut and amaranth flakes and mix well. Press the mixture into a greased, 9-inch by 13-inch baking pan and bake until golden brown. Cool and cut into bars.

Quickie Danish

These are really delicious. When my son Jacob tasted these, he asked if I planned to use the recipe in this book. I told him I did, and he responded, "Mom, file these under 'I' for IRRESISTIBLE." I can't ask for a better endorsement than that.

While this is not the most nutritious recipe in this chapter, it is really a wonderful treat. They are not as sweet as the bakery version, and you could increase the calcium by adding some of Kirkman's calcium powder if you wanted to. For those following Feingold restrictions, use an acceptable jam for the filling. It also uses Sue Crosby's wonderful Quickie Baking Mix found on page 216. If corn must be avoided, stock up on corn-free jams and jellies at Passover time, when they are widely available.

Ingredients

2 cups Quickie Baking Mix

1/4 cup CF margarine, softened

2 tablespoons sugar

1/3 cup DariFree

1/4 cup preserves, jam or lemon curd

Preheat oven to 450°.

Stir together everything but the preserves. You should have a thick, smooth batter. Drop by tablespoons onto a greased or lined cookie sheet, and use the spoon to shape into nice rounds, about 2 inches apart.

Make a small depression in the center of each round using the back of a wet spoon (I use the back of a melon baller to do this).

Fill each depression with 1/4 teaspoon preserves. Bake for 10-15 minutes or until golden brown. If desired, drizzle icing on top.

Icing

Combine 1/3 cup powdered sugar with 1 tablespoon warm water and 1 teaspoon vanilla. Stir until smooth.

Crockpot Cobbler

Put these ingredients in the crockpot before you go to bed, and a delicious hot breakfast will be waiting for you. A great help on those rushed school mornings. If your child does not tolerate apples, substitute firm-fleshed pears.

Ingredients

4 medium-sized apples, peeled and sliced

1/2 cup dried blueberries (use raisins if blueberries are unavailable)

1/4 cup honey

1 teaspoon cinnamon

2 tablespoons ghee or CF margarine, melted

2 cups granola (see recipe on page 36)

Place fruit and other ingredients in crockpot. Mix well, then cover and cook on low for 7-9 hours (overnight) or on high 2-3 hours. Serve with the milk substitute of your choice.

Granola

*I included a granola recipe in **Special Diets for Special Kids**. Here is a slightly different recipe.*

Ingredients

3 cups puffed rice or corn

3 cups GF cornflakes, slightly crushed (omit if corn is not tolerated)

I cup Ener-G Rice Nuts Cereal

$^1/_2$ cup chopped walnuts

$^1/_2$ cup chopped pecans

$^1/_4$ cup sesame seeds

$^1/_4$ cup macadamia nuts*

I cup unsweetened coconut

$^1/_2$ cup raisins and/or dried cranberries

$^1/_3$ cup safflower oil

$^1/_4$ cup honey or cane syrup

$^1/_4$ cup molasses

I $^1/_2$ teaspoons cinnamon

$^1/_4$ teaspoon salt

Preheat oven to 250°. Coat a large roaster pan with vegetable spray. Add all nuts, seed and cereals.

In a saucepan, combine oil, honey, molasses, cinnamon and salt in a saucepan. Stir over low heat until well combined and uniformly hot.

Pour liquid mixture over dry mixture and mix well to coat. Bake for 2 hours, stirring occasionally. Remove from oven and add dried fruit. Mix to combine, then cool completely before storing in a tightly sealed container.

*Macadamia nuts are well-tolerated by most people, but are very expensive.   Omit, or exchange another nut, if you like.

Crunchy Coffeecake

This recipe comes to me from Sue Crosby, the creator of the wonderful Quickie Baking Mix (see page 216).

Ingredients

Batter

1 beaten egg (or egg replacer)

1/2 cup GF/CF milk

1 cup GF/CF flour

1 teaspoon xanthan gum

1/2 teaspoon salt

1/2 cup sugar

2 tablespoons safflower oil

2 teaspoons GF/CF Baking powder

Topping

1/4 cup brown sugar

1 tablespoon tapioca starch

1/4 cup chopped nuts

1 teaspoon cinnamon

1 tablespoon GF/CF Margarine, melted

Beat batter ingredients together until smooth. Pour into a greased 8 x 8 x 2-inch pan. Mix topping ingredients and sprinkle over top of batter. Bake at 375° for 20-25 minutes. Toothpick in center should pull out clean when done.

Apple-cider Doughnuts

Baked doughnuts are easy to make if you have a doughnut pan. These Teflon-coated pans are readily available at cookware stores, and from mail order companies.

Ingredients:

3 tablespoons sugar

2 cups Hagman featherlite flour (or other light GF flour combination)

1 1/2 teaspoons baking powder

1 1/2 teaspoons baking soda

1/2 teaspoon salt

2 teaspoons ground cinnamon

1 large egg, lightly beaten

1/3 cup packed brown sugar

1/3 cup apple or pear butter

1/3 cup pure maple syrup

1/3 cup apple cider

1/3 cup milk substitute, soured with 1/2 teaspoon cider vinegar

3 tablespoons vegetable oil, preferably safflower

Preheat oven to 400°.

Coat depressions of doughnut pan with nonstick cooking spray and sprinkle with sugar.

In a mixing bowl, whisk together dry ingredients and set aside. In another bowl, whisk together egg, brown sugar, apple butter, maple syrup, cider, sour "milk" and oil.

Add dry ingredients and stir just until moistened. Divide half the batter among the prepared molds, spooning about two generous tablespoons of batter into each mold. Use a knife to spread the batter evenly around each mold.

Bake for 10 to 12 minutes, or until the tops spring back when touched lightly. Loosen edges and turn the cakes out onto a rack to cool. Clean the pan, then re-coat it with oil and sugar. Repeat with remaining batter.

Hash Browns

And what goes better with Egg in the Hole than hash browns? My son will eat potatoes prepared in any way imaginable, but hash browns are a special treat.

Ingredients

3 small potatoes, peeled & diced (or shredded if you prefer)

1 teaspoon lemon juice

1/4 cup onion, grated

3 tablespoons oil

Salt and pepper to taste

2 strips bacon, cooked crisp and crumbled (optional)

Sprinkle lemon juice over potatoes and stir in onion and spices. Heat oil over medium heat, then add potatoes. Cook and turn until brown. Potatoes should be soft enough to cut with a fork. Mix in cooked, crumbled bacon if desired.

Churros

One supermarket in our area carries "Churros" a type of cinnamon-coated French toast stick. They are made with wheat flour.   Jacob, who is not GF, adores them. This recipe allows both my boys to enjoy churros. They make a tasty snack too. If serving for breakfast, you can allow the kids to dip in maple syrup. I have no idea why these are called churros, but being the curious type, I attempted to find out. I still don't know, although I did learn alot about a rare breed of sheep by the same name.

Ingredients

1 1/4 cups hot water

1 1/2 cups Quickie biscuit mix (see recipe page 216)

4 cups oil, for frying

1/2 cup white sugar

1 tablespoon ground cinnamon

Heat oil in a deep fryer or deep frying pan.

In a medium bowl, combine the water and baking mix. Beat for about 3 to 4 minutes, until the mixture becomes spongy and uniform. Using a pastry bag, pipe 5-inch long strips of batter into the hot oil.

For best results, fry only a couple at a time. Cook until golden brown, and then drain on paper towels.

In a small bowl stir together the sugar and cinnamon. Dip fried churros in the sugar to coat. Serve hot.

Banana Muffins

Most children like muffins, and I always say they are easy to adjust. Use different ingredients according to your family's likes and dislikes, including nuts and dried fruits. Add calcium powder (one teaspoon per recipe) if you are trying to increase intake of that mineral. Decrease sweetening as desired too. If your kids are little, think about making these as mini-muffins. Remember, little hands can more easily hold little foods.

Ingredients:

3 ripe bananas, mashed

1/2 cup CF margarine

1/2 cup sugar (or sugar substitute)

2 eggs

2 cups GF flour mix

2 teaspoons xanthan gum

1 teaspoon baking soda

Pinch of salt

1 teaspoon of vanilla

Preheat oven to 350°.

Combine dry ingredients in a medium bowl and set aside.

Beat margarine and sugar in an electric mixer until light and creamy. Beat in eggs, one at a time, and then add vanilla. Add dry ingredients and mix well, then mix in the bananas.

Mini muffins bake for 12-15 minutes or until they test done with a toothpick. Larger muffins will bake longer. This recipe can be used for banana bread, too—bake loaves for 50-60 minutes.

Tangy Citrus Muffins

Brenda-Lee Olson, another writer-cook who keeps a gluten free kitchen, created this delicious recipe. Be sure to join her on-line forum, GF/CF RECIPES. To find it, log on to www.yahoogroups.com.

Brenda says that, if you prefer, instead of juicing the lemons and oranges, you can peel them and put them in the blender to liquefy them and use that mash instead of the fresh squeezed juice. You may have to add a little extra pineapple syrup or water if you do, though.

Ingredients

1 1/2 cups fresh-squeezed lemon and orange juice (combine juices to taste)

1 cup crushed pineapple (drained, but reserve syrup)

1 cup syrup from canned, crushed pineapple

1 cup water

1 cup walnuts, chopped (or other nuts)

3 cups GF flour mix

2 teaspoons baking powder

3 eggs

1/2 cup ground sesame seeds

1/2 cup casein free margarine

1/4 teaspoon stevia powder

Preheat the oven to 400°.

In a small bowl, sift together the flours and other dry ingredients. In a separate bowl, cream margarine with stevia, eggs and citrus juices using hand blender or stand mixer. When mixture reaches the texture of curdled milk, add the dry ingredients and mix well. Stir in the water until mixture has the consistency of thick cake batter. Add in the walnuts (or other desired chopped nuts or seeds) and crushed pineapple. Spoon into the prepared muffin tins.

Bake for 20 - 25 minutes or until center of muffin springs up when pressed lightly with an index finger. Flip the muffins over and cook for another 5 - 10 minutes to insure they are cooked all the way through.

This mixture is also stiff enough that it can be used to make free-form biscuits similar to baking powder biscuits by dropping them by the spoonful onto a prepared cookie or stoneware baking sheet.

Note: If you would like the muffins a little sweeter, you can adjust the amount of stevia to suit your taste. I would not, however, use more than one-half teaspoon unless you are experienced with stevia. It is a powerful sweetener and in this case "less is more."

 If you do not have ground sesame seeds, they may be omitted. Their purpose is mostly to add calcium for those who do not eat dairy. If you do omit them, be sure to increase the flours used and to add a little extra baking powder.

Bran Muffins

This is a very tasty way to get some fiber into your child. Add $^1/2$ cup of raisins if you like.

Ingredients

$^1/2$ cup GF flour mix

1 cup bean flour mix (e.g., Garfava flour from Authentic Foods)

$1^1/2$ cups amaranth flakes (available from Gluten Solutions)

$^1/2$ teaspoon salt

$1^1/4$ teaspoons baking soda

$^1/4$ cup molasses

$^1/2$ cup milk substitute, soured with one tablespoon lemon juice

1 egg, beaten

1 tablespoon ghee, melted

1 teaspoon cinnamon

1 tablespoon ground flax seeds

Preheat oven to 350°.

In a large bowl, combine flours, amaranth, flax seed, salt and baking powder. Add molasses, sour "milk", egg and ghee. Stir to mix. Add raisins or other dried fruit if desired.

Scoop batter into muffin pans sprayed with non-stick spray or lined with muffin papers. Cups should be $^1/3$ to $^3/4$ full.

Bake for 20 minutes or until they test done with a toothpick.

Porridge With a Purpose

Many come to this diet because of gastrointestinal problems—in short, their children are constipated! Often parents believe that the opposite is their problem, but Drs. Simon Murch and Andrew Wakefield have shown that ASD kids who seem to have diarrhea often are so constipated that an abdominal x-ray reveals impacted feces. What seems to be diarrhea is the liquid portion that can get around the impaction. Yuck. Not a pretty picture.

For all these kids it is important to promote and maintain what the commercials call "regularity." Here is a recipe that will help. High in fiber and nutritious essential fatty acids, this hot cereal should be a regular on your breakfast table.

Ingredients

1 cup water

2 tablespoons ground flaxseed or Nutriflax powder

2 tablespoons GF hot cereal, uncooked (e.g., Cream of Rice)

Dash of salt

1/2 teaspoon cinnamon

Raisins or other dried fruit (optional)

Sugar or other sweetener, to taste

DariFree or other milk substitute

Bring water and salt to a boil and stir in cereal. Cook over low heat for 1 minute, stirring constantly. Remove from heat and stir in flax, cinnamon and sweetener. Add dried fruit if desired.

Stir in the amount of milk substitute to reach desired consistency and serve.

Crumb Cakes

King Arthur Flour **(www.bakerscatalogue.com)** *sells special paper liners that are perfect for making individual crumb cakes. They are shorter than traditional muffin cups, with a larger diameter. These cakes are like the ones you ate as a child, minus the cellophane wrapping. So don't eye the Drake's Cakes*® *longingly the next time you find them in the local 7-Eleven. Now you can make them yourself. This recipe will make 9 crumb cakes.*

Ingredients

Cake:

1/2 cup CF margarine

I cup sugar

3 eggs

I 1/2 cups GF flour (use a light flour such as Hagman's Featherlite)

2 teaspoons xanthan gum

I 1/3 teaspoons baking soda

3/4 teaspoon salt

1/2 cup soy yogurt (use soured milk substitute if soy is not tolerated)

I 1/3 teaspoons lemon oil

I teaspoon vanilla

Streusel Topping:

3 tablespoons CF margarine

3 tablespoons shortening

3/4 cup GF flour

6 tablespoons brown sugar

3/4 teaspoon cinnamon

1/3 teaspoon salt

Preheat oven to 350°.

In a medium bowl, beat together the margarine and sugar for 2 minutes. Add the eggs, beating well after adding each one, then beat for a total of 5 minutes at medium speed.

Sift together flours, baking soda, salt and xanthan gum. In a separate bowl, combine the yogurt (or sour "milk") with the vanilla and lemon oil.

Stir the dry ingredients into the margarine mixture, alternating with the yogurt and ending with the flour. Place nine crumb cake or regular muffin cups on a cookie sheet. Spoon about 1/4 cup of batter into each cup.

In the food processor, combine all the streusel ingredients until just crumbly (don't let it form a ball). Set aside.

Bake the cakes for about 15 minutes, or until they just look set on top. Remove them from the oven and sprinkle the streusel on top. Work quickly, so that the cakes are returned to the oven as soon as possible. Bake for another 15 minutes or until a toothpick tests clean.

Toaster Corncakes

Here is another use for those special crumb cake papers. (Can you tell I just love these?) If your child cannot tolerate corn (and many cannot) substitute Cream of Rice cereal for the cornmeal.

Ingredients

1 1/2 cups GF flour mix

3/4 cup cornmeal

2 teaspoons xanthan gum

2 1/4 teaspoons baking powder

6 tablespoons sugar (or other sweetener)

3 eggs

2/3 cup milk substitute

1/2 cup CF margarine, melted

Preheat oven to 350°.

In a large mixing bowl, whisk together the GF flour, cornmeal, baking powder, xanthan gum, salt and sugar.

In a separate bowl, combine the eggs and "milk" until well combined (you can do this in the blender if you like). Pour the egg mixture and the melted margarine over the dry ingredients. Stir just to combine.

Place nine muffin cups on a baking sheet and scoop about 1/4 to 1/3 cup of batter into each. Wet your fingers and spread the batter to cover the bottom of the cups. Smooth the tops.

Bake for about 18 minutes or until the bottoms are golden brown but the tops are not. You don't want to over bake because the cakes will be toasted. Allow to cool for 15 minutes before removing from cups.

Hot Cereal Mix

I love to have mixes around the kitchen, but of course those little packets of instant oatmeal and wheat cereals are not in our pantry. This recipe will allow you to keep your own mixture around for quick, hot breakfasts.

Ingredients

5 cups thin cut Poha (rice flakes, available at Indian markets or from Miss Roben's)

1/4 cup brown sugar

3 tablespoons DariFree or Soy milk powder

1 cup raisins (or other dried fruit)

Combine these ingredients and store in an airtight container.

To make cereal, place 1/2 cup of mixture in a bowl. Add 1/4 to 1/2 cups boiling water (adjust the water to the desired consistency). Cereal will thicken in a few minutes.

Peanut Butter Bread

This makes a nice change of pace, anytime. One of my children is really not a breakfast eater and often eats only a small slice of toast or quick bread. I like to use one like this, because it does have some protein. Feel free to use other nut butters if you avoid peanuts.

Ingredients

2 cups GF flour (sorghum or a bean blend would be best)

1/2 cup sugar

2 teaspoons baking powder

1 teaspoon salt

3/4 cup nut butter (I prefer crunchy)

1 large egg

1 cup milk substitute (try almond milk for this)

Preheat oven to 350°.

Combine dry ingredients and then add nut butter. Mix until a crumbly but consistent texture is reached. In a separate bowl, beat together egg and milk and then add to the two nut mixture. Mix until smooth.

Pour batter into a greased loaf pan, or into greased muffin tins. Bake for approximately 1 hour or until bread tests done. Muffins will take about 25 minutes.

Hot Granola

If you like your hot cereal a little crunchier, try using a GF granola. This works best in a microwave, so it's super fast and dirties just the bowl you are serving from.

Ingredients

1/3 cup GF granola (see recipe, page 36)

1/2 cup milk substitute

Combine granola and "milk" in a microwave safe bowl. Cook on high for 2 minutes, or until the cereal starts to boil. Remove from microwave and let stand 1-2 minutes. Stir well before serving.

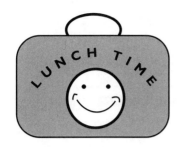

Chapter 4
Lunchbox Favorites

It is hard enough to think of nutritious lunches and snacks for children who have no dietary restrictions, but it is much harder when your child cannot eat some of the old lunchtime standards. Some children prefer a monotonous diet of peanut butter sandwiches, but even the lucky moms (and dads) of those children hate sending in the same fare day after day.

So how do you handle lunch? Perhaps the best tip about lunchtime is this: relax— it's just a meal! Leftovers make great lunches and many school cafeterias have microwaves for reheating meals. You can always heat food in the morning and place it in an insulated container such as a Thermos®. (The Gluten Free Pantry sells a thermal container that has no glass, an important point when you see how your kids toss their backpacks around.) Food stays hot for hours and since many of our kids prefer a hot lunch to a sandwich, this may be a good option.

I have sent in pasta, leftover Chinese food, rice pilaf, chili, stew and even soup. My potato-loving child often takes a spud for lunch—I simply cook it (in the microwave) while he eats his breakfast and then pack it in an insulated container with a little Spectrum spread and salt. It may be Sam's all-time favorite lunch. A Thermos® will keep food cold, too, so you could send in potato salad, cold pasta salads or anything else your child likes to eat.

If your child prefers breakfast to other meals, you can use these foods to make a nutritious lunch that will actually be eaten. Muffins are great lunchbox additions, and if your child loves waffles but hates GF bread, use them for sandwiches. Some kids love left-over pancakes—if yours does make extra the next time you make a pancake breakfast.

The next day, spread a little nut butter and perhaps some jam on 2 or 3 pancakes and roll them up tightly. If they won't stay rolled, use a toothpick to hold them together. They are fun to eat and very nutritious.

When considering what to do about school lunches, take a minute to study the ubiquitous "Lunchable®" in your store's refrigerator case. These ready-made school lunches are low on nutrition and high on price, but kids love them. Why? Obviously, the trick is in the packaging. Another thing that attracts kids to them is that the foods are in appropriately small servings (we often tend to give our kids adult portions). If you think your child would find it appealing, create your own Lunchable®, cutting GF/CF lunchmeats into cubes or small circles. Add just two GF crackers, not a whole stack. Include a fruit and perhaps a few carrot sticks if your child likes crunch. Add two small cookies or an Imagine® brand pudding snack and you've got a lunch your child might actually eat. After all, it doesn't matter how nutritious a meal is if it gets thrown away. Try to get some protein into every meal too—most children do not get enough protein in a typical day.

Let your child's tastes be your guide, and don't feel constrained to pack (or serve) foods specifically created for lunches. Because sandwiches are so often the traditional lunch choice, I have included some bread recipes here.

Since the emphasis in this book is "fast and easy" you may wish to stick to store-bought GF bread, but I hope you will try some of the suggestions in this chapter.

Chicken and Vegetable Chowder

I'm not sure what makes a soup a chowder, but this is a good one no matter what you decide to call it. If your child cannot eat corn, you can use other vegetables. Chowders are usually thickened with cream, but this recipe uses mashed potato flakes. Be sure to buy flakes that are sulfite and additive free (available at health food stores).

Ingredients

6 strips of bacon, cooked

2 tablespoons safflower oil (or bacon fat)

1 medium onion, diced

2 cloves garlic, minced

2 cups cooked chicken, diced

4 cups coconut milk

28 ounces GF chicken broth

1 1/2 cups mashed potato flakes (sulfite-free)

2 cups fresh or frozen corn*

2 cups fresh or frozen mixed vegetables*

Salt, pepper to taste

1 sprig of fresh basil, chopped, or 1/2 teaspoon dried

Cook bacon until crisp; reserve fat and set aside.

In stewpot or Dutch oven, cook onion and garlic in fat. Onions should be soft but not browned. Add all other ingredients and cook for 20 minutes over medium heat.

*Fresh corn or other vegetables may be used. If your child will not eat anything recognizable as a vegetable, thaw and puree the vegetables before adding them to the pot.

NOTE: For vegetarian chowder, omit the chicken and use vegetable broth instead of chicken broth.

Chicken Rice Soup

Even really little kids like chicken rice soup. There is no reason it has to come from a can, which can be pretty sorry stuff. Canned soups often contain many preservatives too. If you have homemade chicken broth this soup is even more delicious, but a good GF canned broth will save time and energy.

Ingredients

1 cup cooked chicken, diced

3 ounces long grain white rice, uncooked

1 carrot, chopped

1/2 cup celery, chopped

1 small potato, peeled and diced

6 cups GF chicken broth

1/2 teaspoon dried parsley

Salt, pepper to taste

Bring the chicken broth to a boil in a large pot. Add all other ingredients and return the soup to a boil. Lower heat, cover and simmer for 10 minutes. Add the rice and stir. Simmer for 15-20 minutes or until the rice is tender.

Potato Soup

There are few things as easy to make as Potato Soup, and it is delicious. When I was a child my mother made this with sour cream, of course, but if your child can tolerate soy, Tofutti Sour Supreme will work just fine. Pureed, it makes a good base for a sauce or casserole.

Ingredients

4 large potatoes, peeled and diced

Water

1 medium onion, diced

1 tablespoon CF margarine

Salt, pepper to taste

3-4 tablespoon mock sour cream

Place potatoes in a pot and add water to just cover them. Add onion and seasoning, and then cook until the potatoes are done (soft), about 20 minutes. Drain all but a little of the water. Add mock sour cream and stir in. You have to "feel" the amount of water—you don't want too much or it the soup will be thin. You want a thick and creamy soup.

Stuffed Apples

Here's another odd one, but it's worth a try for the pickiest of little kids. It has protein and fiber too. If your child cannot tolerate apples, try using a very firm pear.

Ingredients

1 apple (or pear)

Peanut (or other nut) butter

Raisins

Sunflower seeds

Toasted coconut

Core the fruit and stuff with nut butter. Top with as much of the other ingredients as you can fit in. The filling will keep the fruit from turning brown.

Lentil Soup

When Sam was about eight years old, he found that he loved soup. If asked what he wants for dinner, invariably he asks for chili, black bean or lentil soup. Many parents don't introduce soups to their children, assuming that they will not eat it. Remember, most small kids don't like very hot foods, but if the temperature is very warm but not hot, many will eat and enjoy soups. Because most soups can be pureed in a blender or food processor, they are also great for texture sensitive kids. And don't forget to hide the veggies. If needed, puree the vegetables before adding them to the pot.

Ingredients

1 medium onion, chopped

1 cup dry lentils

2 cups GF beef broth (or use water and GF bouillon)

6 cups water

1/2 cup celery, chopped

2 cloves garlic, minced

3 ounces GF pasta (the smallest you can find)

1/4 cup GF spaghetti sauce

1 bay leaf

1 tablespoon fresh parsley, chopped (or one teaspoon dried)

1/2 teaspoon dried thyme

Salt and freshly ground black pepper to taste

Combine broth, water, onion, celery, garlic, tomato sauce, parsley, bay leaf and thyme in a large pot. Bring to a boil.

Rinse the lentils under cold water and drain. Add the lentils to the pot.   Return the pot to boiling, and then lower heat. Cover and let simmer for ^{1}/2 hour.

Add the pasta. Bring to a boil and stir. Lower the heat and simmer for another ^{1}/2 hour, stirring often. If the soup becomes too thick, add a little more water.

Season with salt and pepper to taste.

NOTE: If you prefer, you can substitute ^{1}/2 cup of rice for the pasta, or omit it entirely.

Asian Tenders

My son never tires of chicken tenders (or nuggets). Here is a slightly different take on them, one that your child will like if he or she enjoys the sweet dipping sauces available at some fast food restaurants. The sesame seeds add a nice flavor and a bit of calcium. If you prefer, these can be fried.

Ingredients

1/4 cup orange marmalade (if citrus is a problem, look for pineapple
     marmalade)

1/2 teaspoon ginger

1/4 teaspoon garlic powder

2 tablespoons GF soy sauce (optional)

1 pound chicken tenders, rinsed and dried*

3 cups GF crispy rice cereal, lightly crushed

1/4 cup toasted sesame seeds (optional)

Combine marmalade, ginger, garlic and GF soy sauce in a baking pan (preferably glass). Marinate chicken tenders for at least an hour.

Preheat oven to 400°.

Place sesame seeds in a dry skillet over medium heat, stirring often only until they begin turning golden. Watch them carefully as they can burn quickly. Cool seeds and then combine them with the crushed rice cereal in a pie pan or other low-sided dish.

Dip marinated tenders in the cereal-seed mixture and bake for 10 minutes or until the inside is not pink.

*It is much cheaper to buy chicken breasts and cut your own tenders. Just remove the skin and visible fat, remove the meat from the bone and slice into the size and shape you want. For thin tenders, place meat between sheets of wax paper and pound with a meat mallet. Baking time will vary, depending on how thin or thick you slice the tenders.

PB and Peach Sandwich

If your child loves peanut butter and jelly or jam, but is off sugar, try this slightly odd sandwich. My sister came up with the concept of a peach sandwich when she was on a very strict low-sugar diet. I know it sounds silly, but don't laugh until you've tried it. Children eat lots of things stranger than this (I once went on a pickle relish sandwich binge when I was a kid). And of course, if your child cannot eat peanuts, there are dozens of other nut butters to try.

Ingredients

GF bread or roll (particularly good with GF English muffins)

1 peach, very ripe

Nut butter

Spread slices of bread with nut butter, then top with peeled, ripe peach. If you want to make the peach more like jam, mash and drain it before topping the nut butter.

Gluten Free Spring Rolls

Most kids like foods that they can pick up and eat with their hands, and this recipe makes a really great finger food. The filling can be varied to suit your own needs. The filling below is a traditional egg roll type of filling. You can use what you like. Don't be afraid because these contain vegetables your child won't typically eat. Somehow, when they are wrapped in a spring roll kids do like them. When buying spring roll wrappers be sure you get the ones containing only rice, water (and perhaps salt). They will be round and brittle; the soft wrappers contain wheat flour. You will probably have to go to an Asian market for these, though I can often find them in the ethnic aisle of one of our larger supermarkets.

Filling:

Shredded cabbage

Bamboo shoots (canned), chopped (optional)

Chopped onion or scallion

Shredded, cooked chicken

Mushrooms, chopped

GF Broth

GF Soy Sauce

Garlic

Ginger

Preheat oven to 400°.

Cook the cabbage and mushrooms in a little broth. Then add in the other ingredients.

Cook until the vegetables are soft and the "sauce" thickens a bit.

To use, dip each wrapper separately in a bowl of hot water. It will soften in less than a minute. Remove and fill with about two tablespoons of filling. Wrap up like an envelope, use water to seal edges if necessary.

Place rolls on greased cookie sheet and spray the tops with vegetable spray. Bake for about 10 minutes then turn and bake another 5 minutes or until they are brown and crispy. These are really delicious!

Note: It is tempting to fry these but do not. The skins are too delicate to hold up to frying, and they will fall apart and leave you with a nasty, inedible mess.

Variation: Fill these with a fruit pie filling and sprinkle with a little confectioner's sugar (optional) for dessert.

Ersatz Yogurt

Many of our children love yogurt, and it is a good source of calcium. Alas, once dairy goes, so too goes the yogurt. There are soy alternatives, but many children can't (or won't) eat those. Several years ago Lynne Davis came up with an ingenious recipe for making "yogurt" from DariFree. While it does not contain the live cultures found in real yogurt, kids who miss their Dannon® will enjoy it. (You can supplement with a probiotic.) If your child likes "fruit on the bottom" you can make your own. Mix with fruit in a blender, if that is how your child prefers it. Add GF flavors (e.g., vanilla) as desired.

Ingredients

3/4 cup dry DariFree

3/4 cup unsweetened pineapple juice

1/4 cup lemon juice

2 1/2 cups water

1/2 cup water mixed with 14 teaspoons tapioca starch

Heat juice until hot but not boiling (90 seconds in microwave) and combine with DariFree.

Mix well to dissolve DariFree. Pour mixture into a bowl and add the 2 1/2 cups water.

Heat in microwave for 4-5 minutes until very hot but not boiling. Stir in the last 1/2 cup water mixed with the tapioca starch. It should thicken up immediately as you stir. If not, heat another minute or so until it begins to thicken, stirring often to prevent lumps.

Cool in the fridge for 24 hours. If you use it sooner it will be gummy. Add fruit or jam or use as a dressing for fruit salad. Stir it into fruit at the last minute as it will separate in a few hours if used as a dressing.

Potato Logs

Dedicated GF/CF mom Lisa Ackerman contributed this recipe for potato logs, and promises your child will like them. That's because if her son Jeff likes them, she is fairly sure that any kid will eat them. Lisa insists that he is the world's pickiest child, but then, I bet you think your child wins that award. Jeff says "two enthusiastic thumbs up."

Ingredients

4 large white potatoes (cooked and grated)

2 medium sized yellow squash (grated but not cooked)

1/4 cup ghee or GF/CF margarine

Sea salt and pepper to taste

Preheat oven to 425°.

Combine grated potatoes and squash with melted ghee or margarine. Season with salt and pepper and mix well. (Mixing with your hands may work best.)

Form into little logs (no longer than the size of your palm) and place on ungreased cookie sheet. Bake for 25 minutes or until golden brown.

Oven Fries

This is an easy way to cook "fries" if you are cutting back on fat. Some children will only eat potatoes that are actually fried, but most will accept oven-fried potatoes too.

Ingredients

2 pounds potatoes

1 tablespoon oil (olive or safflower)

1 tablespoon paprika

Sea salt to taste

Preheat the oven to 425°.

Wash the potatoes well and peel, if you wish. In a large bowl, stir together the oil and paprika and set aside.

Cut the potatoes lengthwise into 1/2 inch strips. Toss the potatoes in the oil and spices until well coated. Arrange the potatoes in a single layer on a baking sheet lightly oiled. Bake 45 to 60 minutes, stirring occasionally, until the fries are golden and crisp. Sprinkle with salt to taste and serve.

Joya's Potato Nuggets

I met Joya Sabouni after a talk I gave in Souderton, Pennsylvania. She kindly sent me a few of her son's favorite recipes and I'm happy to share them with you. My son absolutely adores potatoes, and will eat them in virtually any form. It gets boring always serving fries; here is a nice change of pace kind of recipe, and one that uses vegetables and eggs.

Ingredients

6 medium potatoes

1 onion, chopped

1-2 eggs

6 ounces frozen, chopped spinach (thawed)

Preheat oven to 375°.

Boil the potatoes until tender, then peel and quarter them and squeeze them through a potato ricer*.

Add the chopped onion and one egg. Squeeze as much water as possible out of the spinach and add to the potato mixture. Add the second egg if needed to achieve a texture that can be formed into small nuggets. Add salt and pepper if desired.

Shape into nuggets with spoons or moistened hands, and bake on a greased cookie sheet until crispy and golden brown. Turn once so both sides are golden. These can also be fried if you prefer.

*See glossary

Meat Puffs

*Lisa Ackerman modified a recipe from **Special Diets for Special Kids** to make this tasty little item. Her son swears by it. She says that this recipe has helped even the fussiest kids eat protein and veggies, and suggests starting with 1/4 cup vegetables, then increasing to at least a cup over time. It's a good way to use up leftover meat or chicken.*

Ingredients

14 ounces meat (pork, turkey, or chicken), cooked

1/2 cup GF Breading* (use a food processor or coffee grinder to make
    breading fine)

1 egg, or egg replacement substitute equivalent to one egg

1/2 cup water or milk substitute

1 1/2 teaspoons GF/CF baking powder

Salt and pepper to taste

1 teaspoon Flaxseed powder (optional)

1/4 cup - 1 cup cooked vegetables (blended)

Preheat oven to 350°.

Puree meat with just enough water to make a paste.

Put all ingredients into bowl. Mix well. Make meat puffs into little balls or logs. Place balls on lightly greased baking sheet. Cook 18-25 minutes until light brown.

*Lisa rotates her son's foods, so she uses quinoa flakes and quinoa flour one day, GF crispy rice cereal and rice flour on other days, and potato flour and potato buds on potato days. Miss Roben's breading mix would be another good choice.

Buckwheat Bread

*I am always thrilled to get a recipe from Lynne Davis. She has created so many good ones, including the original Pineapple Velvet Cake in **Special Diets for Special Kids**. This recipe makes nice dark bread with a great flavor. You can also use it for pizza dough.*

Ingredients

1/2 cup very warm water

1 tablespoon yeast

1 teaspoon sugar

1 1/3 cups brown rice flour or GF blend

3/4 cups buckwheat flour

1/2 cup tapioca starch

1 tablespoon xanthan gum

1 1/4 cups ground almonds or almond flour

2 eggs, beaten

1 teaspoon apple cider vinegar

1/4 cup brown sugar

1 teaspoon salt

1 1/4 cups soy milk or DariFree

1/3 cup oil

Preheat oven to 375°

Start with all ingredients at room temperature (except the water). Combine yeast with warm water and sugar.

Combine dry ingredients and set aside. Put remaining ingredients in large mixer bowl and mix well. Add in the yeast mixture, then the dry ingredients and mix well. Put into oiled pans, either two 9 x 5-inch pans or 4 mini loaf pans. Cover and let rise in a warm place for 30 minutes. Bake for 35 to 40 min.

Potato wrap

Here is another of Joya Sabouni's recipes. This works well for wrap-type sandwiches. It is similar to a pita, and is a useful recipe for people who are using rotation diets.

        2 cups mashed potatoes

        I cup GF/CF flour

        I teaspoon salt

Combine mashed potatoes with flour and salt. Work together until it forms a dough.

Transfer dough to counter and shape into a long rope. Slice the dough into one-inch sections. Roll the slices of dough into round circles, the size of a tortilla or pita.

Heat a heavy, dry frying pan on top of the burner. When the pan is very hot, put in a flat bread circle. Cook until dough blisters and begins to brown. Turn. Finish cooking the other side. When all of them are done, brush with melted margarine or ghee (optional).

Use like a pita and wrap your favorite filling.

Yeast-Free Sorghum Bread

Kelly Weaver is the source of this terrific bread. Sorghum flour (sometimes called Jowar or Juwar) is a wonderful addition to the GF kitchen. It works well in recipes developed for wheat flour and gives those who rotate an additional choice. It is now fairly easy to find at the health food store.

This recipe is special because it is hard to find a good yeast free bread that slices and tastes like the real thing.

Ingredients

2 cups sorghum flour

1 $^1/_2$ teaspoons xanthan gum

$^1/_2$ teaspoon GF/CF baking soda

2 teaspoons GF/CF baking powder

2 teaspoons dried egg whites

$^1/_2$ teaspoon salt

2 eggs (can use egg replacer if necessary)

3 tablespoons shortening* (Spectrum palm shortening or ghee or GF/CF
   margarine or oil)

2 tablespoons honey

1 cup plus one tablespoon soda or sparkling water

Preheat to oven 350°.

Combine all ingredients and mix well. Consistency will be like cake batter. Grease and flour (with spectrum and sorghum) a bread pan.

Bake 30 min. Cover with foil and bake 25 min. longer. Remove from pan and cool.

*Spectrum now makes a trans-fat-free solid shortening that can be used in place of Crisco® or other hard shortenings. You could also use ghee, GF/CF margarine or even oil in this recipe.

Deviled Eggs

If eggs are tolerated they are a terrific source of protein. Many kids who wouldn't dream of touching a plain egg will eat a deviled one. If you can, pipe the filling through a pastry tube. They look so appetizing when made this way that even a fussy little one may be induced to try them.

Ingredients

6 eggs, hard-boiled

1/4 cup GF mayonnaise

1/2 teaspoon mustard

1/4 teaspoon GF Worcestershire sauce

1 teaspoon sweet pickle relish (optional)

Salt and pepper to taste

Paprika (optional for garnish)

Cut eggs in half lengthwise. Remove yolks. Mash with a fork, and mix with the remaining ingredients. Mound or pipe mixture into egg whites. Sprinkle with paprika.

Squash Latkes

Latkes (pancakes) are traditionally made from potatoes. My friend Randee found herself with some extra spaghetti squash last summer, and got the bright idea of using it to make latkes. Her vegetable-phobic children had no idea what they were eating and gobbled them right down.

Ingredients

and removed from skin with a fork

lol-Grain rice crackers) or breading

microwave is the easiest way to cook it. To
ife (this is important—if not pierced in sev-
ok on high until it is tender when pressed
ites depending on the size of the squash
microwave does not have a turntable,

Let squ　　　　　　　　　　　　ou can handle it easily. Cut it in half
and rem

Using the tines of a fork, scrape out the flesh of the squash. It will come out in spaghetti-like strands. Place the squash in a large bowl and add the eggs, salt and enough of the crumbs so that the mixture is stiff enough to form into patties.

Heat oil for a few minutes, then form latkes with wet hands and fry until golden and crispy on all sides.

Note: spaghetti squash has a pleasant, mild flavor. When served with marinara sauce many children will eat it. You may also want to toss it with some CF margarine or a little melted ghee. Add salt and serve as a side dish.

Buckwheat Pete's Honey-Buckwheat Pitas

Peter De Niverville (aka "Buckwheat Pete") has published an e-book that can be purchased online, downloaded and read or printed via Adobe Acrobat® software.

In the book, Buckwheat Pete Bakes Pitas & Tea Biscuits, Pete presents an unusual bread-making technique. It involves cooking tapioca starch until it is sticky and opaque, and then gently kneading it into the GF flour mixture. The cooked tapioca starch provides the binding and stretchiness that usually come from xanthan or guar gum. Because xanthan gum is derived from corn, there may be some extremely sensitive corn intolerant people who cannot use it (though the vast majority can). Further, xanthan gum is very expensive and even though it is used in small amounts it may be worth your while to experiment with Pete's method.

*Go to **www.buckwheatpete.com** for information on ordering his electronic book. For rice pitas, merely substitute white rice flour for buckwheat flour. These pitas form a strong pocket for stuffing with your child's favorite sandwich filler.*

Ingredients

1 1/2 cups light buckwheat flour

1/2 cup tapioca starch plus 1 1/2 cups warm water

1 tablespoon honey

1/2 teaspoon salt

1/4 cup sunflower oil

2 teaspoons dried chives (optional)

Preheat oven to 375°.

In a large mixing bowl combine the flour, salt and chives (if desired)

Add the honey and oil and blend with a pastry blender until the mixture is grainy. Form a well in the middle of the flour mixture and set aside.

Dissolve the tapioca starch flour with the warm water in a large, microwave-proof glass measuring cup. Microwave on high for 2-3 minutes, stirring twice, or until the mixture has thickened and becomes clear and sticky. It should look like petroleum jelly, but will be thicker and stickier. There must be no liquid left in the tapioca mixture or the tapioca will not bind with the flour. Allow the mixture to cool.

Place the cooked tapioca in the well you made in the flour mixture. Knead by hand until all the flour has disappeared into the mixture.*   Form the dough into a ball. Divide the ball into four pieces and form each into a patty.

On a GF floured surface, roll out each patty to $1/8$ to $1/4$ inch thickness. Use a spatula to transfer to a non-stick baking sheet. Bake for 15-18 minutes or until slightly browned. Put on a wire rack to cool and cover with a clean dishtowel.

*Kneading in all the flour mixture will take a little elbow grease, but don't give up. You will be rewarded with smooth, workable dough.

Indian Fry Bread

My parents have begun spending winters in Scottsdale, Arizona, and last winter we were lucky enough to visit them in February. Everything was new and different, and I noticed that everywhere we went there were stands that sold "fry bread." It turned out that they are relatively easy to make with GF flours. Simpler to make than donuts (and with a lot less sugar) this is a delicious addition to a lunch or breakfast table.

Ingredients

3 cups GF flour mix

1 tablespoon baking powder

1/2 teaspoon salt

2 teaspoon xanthan gum

1 1/2 cups warm water

1/2 cup raisins or other dried fruit (optional)

Honey or GF rice syrup

Oil, for frying

Combine dry ingredients in a bowl. Add warm water in small amounts and knead dough until soft but not sticky. Adjust flour or water as needed. Cover bowl and let stand about 30 minutes.

Heat oil to about 350°. Pull off pieces of dough the size of an egg. Roll out into 1/4 inch rounds and about 5 inches in diameter. With a knife, cut a whole in the center of each round (so that they will fry flat). Fry the rounds in hot oil until the first side is golden brown, then turn and fry on the other side until it's the same color as the first.

For breakfast, brush with honey on top and serve while warm. For lunch, use your favorite toppings or make a Native American "taco": top with chili and soy cheese first, then cover with lettuce and tomatoes, onions and green chilis.

Rice Dogs

Here is a "corn dog" for the corn-intolerant. It uses a Cream of Rice® type cereal. These really taste good with the added sugar, but go ahead and try it without if you must avoid it. This is a great treat for parties and picnics.

Ingredients

2 cups GF flour blend

3/4 cup Cream of Rice®*

1/4 cup sugar

2 teaspoons salt

3/4 cup milk substitute

2 egg yolks, beaten slightly

8 hot dogs**

8 cups oil

Wooden skewers or chopsticks

Preheat oil to 375° in a deep pan or fryer.

Combine the dry ingredients in one bowl, and milk and eggs in another. Then combine all together and beat with electric mixer until you have a thick, smooth batter.

Skewer the hot dogs, and dip carefully in the batter. Cover the dogs on all sides and let excess batter drip off. The dogs will coat more evenly if you dry them with paper towels first.

Hold the sticks and carefully submerge each dog in the oil. Turn the stick slowly so that the coating cooks evenly. After 20 seconds or so you can let go of the skewer, which will enable you to make more than one at a time. Cook each dog for 5 minutes or until the coating turns a dark golden brown. Turn the dogs once or twice as they cook. Drain on paper towels.

* Cream of Rice® cereal contains only granulated rice, but it is made in a plant that also makes wheat products. I have never had a problem with this product, but if you prefer, there are health food store versions that carry no risk of cross contamination. Always call manufacturers if you are unsure.

**Always take care (read labels!) when buying hot dogs. Many contain milk products: there are Kosher dogs available that do not. You may prefer to buy the hot dogs that contain no preservatives at all—check the freezer section of your health food store. These must be kept frozen until cooked. Many of the chicken and turkey dogs are also acceptable but again, read the labels carefully.

Franks-in-Blankets

This recipe comes to me from Nadine Gilder. Be sure to make a bunch of these in advance and freeze them, taking them out when you're ready to use them.

For more of Nadine's recipes, you can purchase her booklet "Gluten- and Casein-Free Cooking: Recipes for Everyday Favorites." Send a check or money order for $8 plus $3 shipping and handling to: Nadine Gilder/1218 Steeplechase Court/Toms River, NJ 08755.

Ingredients

3 1/2 cups GF flour mix

1 tablespoons xanthan gum

1 1/2 teaspoons salt

3/4 cup sugar

3 eggs

1 teaspoon GF vinegar

4 tablespoons oil

1 cup warm water (not hot)

1 tablespoon GF yeast

1 package GF/CF frankfurters

Preheat oven to 350°

In a small bowl, combine the warm water; add the yeast and one teaspoon of the sugar. Make sure that yeast is dissolved. Mix and let stand for 5 minutes to proof. (It should be foamy after 5-10 minutes—if it is not, use fresh yeast.)

Next, add the first four ingredients to a larger mixing bowl and stir well.

Add yeast mixture to the flour and then add the eggs, vinegar and oil.

Beat dough with electric mixer, or use the "dough" cycle of your bread machine. Beat until all ingredients are well blended, then place the dough in a lightly oiled bowl, cover with a clean, damp towel and let it stand in a warm place until it has doubled in size. Check often to make sure it does not rise over the bowl.

Wrap the Frankfurters

Turn dough out onto a GF floured board or countertop. If too sticky to handle, add a little GF flour to it and knead by hand. Take a softball-sized piece of dough and roll it out flat to a thickness of about 1/4-inch.

Next, place the frankfurters on the dough, one at a time and roll them up. (For less bread, use a smaller piece of dough.) The more layers of dough you wrap around, the thicker the bread around the frankfurter will be. Use a moistened finger to seal the edge of the dough.

Place the wrapped franks (whole or cut) onto a greased tin and bake for 20 minutes or until the dough is golden brown. Serve, or cool and freeze and reheat later.

NOTE: You can freeze the wrapped, unbaked franks. If baking later, you will need to increase baking time by a few minutes.

Chicken Quiche

Brown rice makes a nice "crust" for this quiche. Add vegetables to this for an even nicer dish, if you think you can get your kids to eat them. This quiche cuts into nice wedges that could even be picked up without too big a mess.

Ingredients

1 1/2 cups water

3/4 cup brown rice

1 small summer squash

1 cup cooked chicken, cut into small cubes

1 teaspoon prepared minced garlic

1 small onion, diced

Vegetable oil spray

1 egg white

1/4 teaspoon salt

2 eggs

1 cup evaporated milk (see recipe on page 213)

Salt and pepper, to taste

Preheat oven to 450°.

Place water in a small saucepan. Bring to a boil over high heat. Add rice and stir. Return to boiling. Reduce heat and simmer, covered, for 35 to 40 minutes, or until rice is tender and liquid is absorbed.

Chop squash and combine with onion and garlic. Sauté over medium heat until tender but not mushy. Add chicken and mix well. Set aside.

In a small mixing bowl, stir together cooked rice, egg white, and 1/4 teaspoon salt. Press mixture onto the bottom and up the sides of a quiche dish or pie pan. Bake, uncovered, for 5 minutes. Remove from oven and reduce oven temperature to 325°.

In a medium mixing bowl, stir together eggs, evaporated "milk", 1/4 teaspoon salt, and pepper. Spoon chicken mixture into the crust, and then carefully pour egg mixture on top.

Bake for 35 to 40 minutes, or until a knife inserted near the center comes out clean. Let stand 10 minutes before cutting.

Mock Runzas®

Growing up in Omaha, Nebraska, I spent many Saturday afternoons at the University of Nebraska's Memorial Stadium. That's right—college football. As the season progresses, it gets really, really cold in the stadium, and sandwiches from the Runza Hut® stand not only tasted great, but also served as hand warmers. Wrapped in foil, we held on to them as long as we could stand it. Usually we ate them before too long because they smelled great and it was just too tempting. I've never seen Runzas® in the east, but they are still available back home.

Of course, they call for wheat flour and yeast, but you can make a tasty Runza® knock-off using Miss Roben's GF pizza mix. Besides being delicious, these contain cabbage but your kids won't know it. Combine leftover filling with cooked GF noodles for another quick dinner.

Ingredients

1 pound ground beef

1/2 head cabbage, shredded

3 onions, very thinly sliced

1/2 teaspoon garlic powder

1 package Miss Roben's GF Pizza Crust mix

5 tablespoons sugar (optional)

1 egg, beaten with one tablespoon water

Preheat oven to 375°.

Brown beef and remove from pan; sauté onions in the hamburger fat until soft. Add cabbage and cook until the vegetables are very soft. Return the cooked beef to the pan and add approximately 1/2 cup water. Continue cooking until the cabbage and onions are very, very soft. Add more water as needed and cook until tender, adding a little water if it gets too dry. Season with garlic powder, salt and pepper.

Prepare pizza dough mix according to package directions. Use as little water as possible so that the dough will be easy to roll out. If using the optional sugar, add it to the dry mix. Be sure to use the yeast packets that come with the dough mix.

To form sandwiches, break off an egg-sized piece of dough and roll out on a GF flour covered surface, to a 4" square or circle. The Runza® sandwich is rectangular, but you can make a more traditional meat turnover by folding a circular piece of dough in half.*

Place 1-2 tablespoons meat filling in the dough; the amount you use will depend on how large the dough is. Be sure to pinch the edges firmly to seal. Use a little water if needed for a tight seal—you don't want the filling to leak out. Brush with beaten egg wash and bake for 20 minutes or until the turnovers are golden brown.

*I bought a "pot sticker mold" for under $5 at a kitchenware store. This little plastic mold is hinged; you place a small circle of dough on it, spoon on a teaspoon of filling, then close the mold. *Voila!* Perfectly formed little meat pies. You could also use a ravioli maker—roll out the dough in strips to fit the mold, fill each cavity with meat filling, and place a second strip on top.

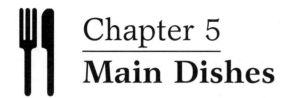

Chapter 5
Main Dishes

*D*inner—why, oh why, is it so hard to come up with fresh ideas? And who has time to actually cook? Our lives are so busy and so stressful that, on many nights, just thinking about dinner can seem like a formidable task.

In this chapter I have tried to come up with lots of ideas for dinner, but beyond that I have tried to emphasize main dishes that are really simple to put together. My goal is to present super-easy recipes that look (and taste) as if they took much more effort than you actually expended.

To accomplish this goal, I have gone back to the past. In the early sixties, the emphasis was on "convenience" foods, and American housewives (face it—that's who was doing the cooking back then) loved them. Women's magazines were filled with recipes that could be put together quickly, often using bottled and canned foods.

These foods, and the recipes they spawned, were easy. Problem is, they weren't all that nutritious. They generally relied on over-processed versions of real food. Many of the basic ideas were solid though, and I've used some of them to create some modern, healthful dinners. Many of the ingredients are available at health food stores, and my recipes use more fresh ingredients than the original versions. If you are as old as I am, I bet some of these will ring a distant bell.

Lillian's Chicken

I don't know who Lillian is, but when my good friend Randee Tengi gave me this recipe she insisted that I retain the name. This tasty chicken dish is so simple you will find yourself making it often when you just don't have time to do anything fancy. Great with rice, this version is a variation of the original recipe. It uses two ingredients commonly found in health food stores.

Ingredients

1 bottle Annie's Naturals® French or Raspberry Vinaigrette salad dressing

1 envelope Fantastic Foods® onion dip/soup mix or use recipe on page 225

1 small can mandarin oranges (in water if possible)

1 pound chicken parts (preferably skinned, boneless breasts)

In blender, process oranges coarsely, leaving a few chunks if desired. Mix with onion soup and salad dressing. Marinate chicken in mixture for an hour or overnight.

Bake at 350° for 1 hour. Serve over rice or GF noodles.

Easiest Chicken and Dumplings

Chicken and dumplings may be one of the greatest "comfort foods" I know of, but it doesn't have to be a big deal to make. This recipe will work well with leftover chicken. If you are really pressed for time, you can buy pre-cooked chicken breast meat. Be sure to check the spices and other ingredients if you go that route.

Ingredients

1 32-ounce container of Imagine® Cream of Potato and Leek soup

1 package of mixed frozen vegetables (your choice)

Shredded Tofutti® or Soymage® soy cheese (optional—use if soy is tolerated)

1 teaspoon arrowroot starch (use if cheese is omitted)

4 large pieces or 6 small pieces of cooked chicken (e.g. 4 breasts)

Heat the soup to boiling in a 4-quart saucepan. Add the vegetables and cook over medium heat until it returns to a boil. Lower to simmer and cook for about 10 minutes (the exact cooking time will depend on your choice of vegetables and their size). If desired, add 1/2 to 1 cup of soy cheese and cook until melted. Cut chicken into bite size pieces, add to the pot and heat through.

If you do not use the soy cheese, remove about a cup of the liquid from the saucepan and stir the arrowroot starch into the removed liquid. Be sure that all lumps are dissolved, then add the mixture back to the pot. This will thicken the stew.

Dumplings*

   1 cup Gift of Nature® GF Flour mix**

   1 1/2 teaspoons baking powder

   Salt to taste

   2 tablespoons shortening

   1/2 cup milk substitute

Combine flour mix, baking powder and salt in a medium sized bowl. Using a pastry blender or two knives, cut in the shortening until the mix resembles coarse corn meal. Slowly add the milk substitute and mix until you have a soft, thick dough.

With a large spoon or wet hands, form dumplings and place on top of the gently boiling chicken mixture. Cook for 10 minutes uncovered, then cover the pot and cook for an additional 10 minutes.

*If you have a batch of Quickie Dough mix on hand, you can use the recipe on page 216 to make dumplings.

**You can use other GF flour mixes, but this one works particularly well.

Simple Chicken Stew

   *This simple recipe appeared in a 2000 issue of **The ANDI News**. I try not to repeat myself, but it is so good and so easy that I wanted to include it in this book. This stew works well with boned, skinned breast meat and is another comfort food for cold winter nights. Actually, it isn't exactly a recipe because no specific amounts are given. Determine the ingredients you use based on what your family likes. Quantities needed must be based on the amount of meat you are cooking. It's OK to "wing it" when cooking.*

Ingredients

Chicken

Oil

Sweet rice flour (available at Chinese groceries)

Vegetables (your choice)

GF/CF Bouillon

In a heavy skillet at least 3 inches deep, brown chicken in a few tablespoons of oil. If the meat sticks, add some gluten-free chicken stock. While the meat is browning, sprinkle in a few teaspoons of sweet rice flour.

When the meat is browned, add water to cover about 1/3 of the meat. Add a few chopped onions, potatoes, carrots and any other vegetable your family likes. Then add a good gluten and casein free bouillon (available through The Gluten Free Pantry and many other suppliers of GF/CF items). If any lumps form, press them out with the back of a spoon.

Bring to a boil, then lower heat and cover. Simmer the dish for an hour or until the meat is cooked through and the vegetables are tender. If the sauce is not thick enough, simmer uncovered. Add peas, broccoli or other quick cooking vegetables during the last 10 minutes of cooking. If boned meat is used, cut into bite sized chunks when tender.

Note: If your child tolerates soy and can eat fermented foods (i.e., is not on a yeast-free diet) you can substitute miso paste for bouillon. Read the ingredients carefully, as some pastes are made with barley. These pastes are high in protein and extremely flavorful. There are even rice misos available, although they are harder to find. A small "dollop" greatly improves the flavor of a large pot of soup or stew. Miso paste can be found in the refrigerator section of most health food stores.

Easiest Meatballs

Here's another easy dish that originated in the sixties. Both my kids love these meat-balls. You can prepare these on the stove over very low heat, but I sometimes put them in the crockpot in the morning and forget about them until dinnertime. If you cook these on the stove, be sure to keep the heat very low and to check often to prevent burning.

Ingredients

1 pound ground meat (sirloin or ground turkey works best)

1 egg (omit if eggs are not tolerated)

1 8-ounce jar organic grape jam

1 12-ounce GF chili sauce*

GF cracker crumbs, finely ground (I use Hol Grain®)

In slow cooker set on high, combine the jam and chili sauce. Heat until the jam is melted.

Combine ground meat with egg and cracker crumbs until you can form meatballs that hold together. Make small meatballs and place gently in slow cooker.

Set to low. Cook for 3 hours or until done.

*If you cannot find GF chili sauce, add 2 teaspoons of horseradish to 1 1/2 cups of GF catsup.

"Cheesy" Meatballs

These are tasty meatballs, and easy to make if your family tolerates soy. Put the cereal in a Ziploc® type bag, seal it and have your child crush it with a rolling pin. Soymage® makes a delicious Parmesan cheese that, as of this writing, is totally gluten and casein free. If soy is off-limits, these are still good without it.

Ingredients

1 pound lean ground beef (I use sirloin)

1/2 teaspoon salt

1/2 teaspoon garlic powder

Pepper to taste

1/2 cup GF/CF Parmesan

1 egg

1/2 cup Gorilla Munch® cereal, crushed

Spaghetti sauce of your choice

Combine all ingredients except sauce and mix lightly. Form into small balls and brown in a skillet coated lightly with cooking spray. Bring spaghetti sauce to a boil and add meatballs. Simmer for 20 minutes, until meatballs are done.

Serve alone or with spaghetti.

Hawaiian Meatballs

Ok, so I have included a lot of meatball recipes. I'm a big fan of meatballs because most kids, even really picky ones, like them. My son Jake is very fussy, but he loves meatballs of almost any description. This one is sweet, and for some may be the only way to get some protein in the diet.

I hope that at least one of these recipes will suit your family. Remember, you can use any ground meat or combination of meats. On occasion, I even use ground ostrich. Don't use this recipe if you are on a yeast-free diet.

Ingredients

1 cup crispy rice cereal*

1 cup DariFree powder or soy milk powder

1/4 cup onion, minced

1 egg

1 pound lean ground meat

1 15-ounce can GF tomato sauce

1/2 cup GF ketchup

1/4 cup firmly packed brown sugar

1/4 cup crushed pineapple in water, well drained

2 tablespoons GF Worcestershire sauce (optional)

1 tablespoons apple cider vinegar

Salt and pepper (to taste)

Preheat oven to 400°.

Combine cereal, onions, DariFree, egg, 2 tablespoons ketchup, and salt and pepper. Add the meat and mix until well combined. Form meatballs and place in a baking pan coated with cooking spray. Bake for 10-15 minutes or until browned.

Combine the other ingredients in a saucepan, and simmer over low heat for 15 minutes. Add browned meatballs to sauce and cook over low heat for another 15 minutes. Serve with rice or GF noodles.

*As of this writing, New Morning Crispy Rice Cereal® was both GF and very tasty. Always be sure to check and recheck ingredients.

Mini-Meat Loaves

Kids who often turn their noses up at meat loaf will eat it if they have a really small one. Use tiny loaf-sized pans (available at kitchen stores) or muffin tins.

Ingredients

1 1/2 pounds lean ground meat (beef, turkey, chicken)

1 egg, beaten (optional)

8 ounces spaghetti sauce

1/2 cup GF cracker crumbs (Dr. Scharr's crumbs are excellent)

Salt and pepper

Shape into 3-inch balls and cook them in muffin tins at 350° for 30-45 minutes (depending on size). Drain grease before serving with potatoes.

Frito® Pie

These crunchy treats are not the world's most healthful snack, but boy, are they good—and kids love them. They contain too much fat, too much salt and too many preservatives, but as a very occasional snack I guess they cannot do TOO much harm. Both my kids adore them and they are gluten free.

They love this dish, and your kids will too. Kind of retro, but easy and good. If you prefer another chili recipe, feel free to use it, but be sure it is a recipe that isn't too soupy or the casserole will have too much liquid. If you are lucky enough to live near a Trader Joe's store, you will be able to find a corn chip free of all the "junk" (but still full of fat and flavor).

Ingredients

1 pound lean ground beef

1 large onion chopped fine (puree in blender if your child isn't an onion fan)

1 clove garlic, crushed

1 28-ounce can tomatoes

1 teaspoon GF chili powder

1 teaspoon ground cumin

1 teaspoon salt

1 19-ounce can refried beans (preferably fat free)

2 cups Fritos® corn chips (or other brand, preferably additive free)

1 cup GF/CF "cheese," shredded (optional)

Preheat the oven to 350°.

Cook the beef in a skillet, and add the onions and garlic once some fat has been released into the pan. Cook until the meat loses its pink color, and the vegetables are getting soft. Drain excess fat and then add the tomatoes (with juice) and the seasonings.

Simmer for about 30 minutes, and then stir in the refried beans and mix thoroughly.

Cover the bottom of a 9 x 13-inch baking pan with one cup of chips. Cover with chili and GF/CF cheese if desired. Use remaining chips for the top. Bake for 20 minutes.

Baked Kibbe

Kibbe is a middle-eastern dish, sort of a lamb meatloaf. It is usually served with a mint-flavored yogurt sauce, but is delicious even without this forbidden condiment.

Ingredients

1 pound ground lamb

1 tablespoon onion, minced

1/2 teaspoon ground allspice

1/4 teaspoon cumin

1/2 teaspoon ginger

1 egg

1 teaspoon minced parsley

1/2 teaspoon salt

3 tablespoons GF breadcrumbs (or cooked rice)

2 cloves garlic, crushed

Preheat oven to 375°.

Combine all ingredients and shape into 8 small loaves. Bake in a 9-inch dish for 20 minutes or until browned. Serve with rice pilaf.

Super-Simple Shepherd's Pie

Special Diets for Special Kids included a recipe for Shepherd's Pie, and it remains a favorite at our house. However, there are times when you just have to take a shortcut or two. Frozen mixed vegetables really work well in this recipe, and Bird's Eye® has some wonderful new combinations called "Farm Fresh Selections." A good GF/CF salsa is another good addition.

If you're in a hurry go ahead and use instant mashed potatoes—just be sure to get sulfite-free potato flakes (available at some groceries and at health food stores).

Ingredients

I tablespoon safflower oil

I pound lean ground meat

I onion, chopped very fine

I clove garlic, minced

I pound bag of mixed frozen vegetables

I cup fresh mushrooms, chopped fine (omit if on yeast-free diet)

I cup GF salsa

4 cups mashed potatoes (prepared)

Salt and pepper (to taste)

Preheat oven to 350°.

Heat oil in a skillet, then cook onion, garlic until soft. Add mushrooms and cook until mushrooms give up their liquid, then add the meat. Continue cooking over medium heat, until the meat is cooked through. Add vegetables and return the pot to boiling.

Add salsa and cook for an additional 10 minutes. Season with salt and pepper, then pour mixture into a casserole.

Top with mashed potatoes and bake the casserole for 35-40 minutes, until the top is golden and the meat is bubbling.

Mexican Cornbread Pizza

This is a simple recipe that is very easy to throw together. If your child cannot tolerate corn, you can substitute Cream of Rice® cereal for cornmeal in this recipe. If soy isn't tolerated, there really are no good cheese alternatives; you may wish to call it something else so that cheese is not expected.

Ingredients

1 recipe cornbread

1 pound ground beef

1 onion, chopped

1 teaspoon chili powder

1 teaspoon garlic powder

1/4 cup salsa

Salt and pepper to taste

1 8-ounce package Tofutti® shredded cheddar style cheese, divided

Preheat oven to 400°.

Prepare cornbread and spread batter into greased 12-inch pizza pan. Bake for 8 to 10 minutes, or until lightly brown.

Brown meat and onion and then drain. Add seasoning to salsa and spoon over crust. Sprinkle 1-cup "cheese" over baked crust. Top with meat mixture and remaining cheese.

Bake 4 to 5 minutes, or until cheese is melted.

Veggie Burgers

Rebecca Sullivan is a mom who wrote to me looking for a play-clay recipe two years ago. When I sent her the recipe that had appeared in The ANDI News, she was so thrilled that she immediately sent me her own recipe for veggie burgers. It has been a big hit with her family, and is a great way to sneak in some lima beans, if you're so inclined.

Ingredients

1/2 pound lima beans, cooked

1 carrot

1 onion

1 apple, cored, peeled and sliced (substitute pear if apples are not tolerated)

2 eggs (or equivalent egg replacer)

1/4 cup tapioca flour

2 tablespoons potato starch

1 teaspoon parsley

1 teaspoon xanthan gum

1/2 teaspoon salt

1/4 - 1/2 cup water for processing

Place all vegetables in the food processor and process. Add eggs and continue to process until smooth.

Add flours and all other ingredients except lima beans and process to incorporate. Add lima beans and process for 2 minutes or until completely mixed. Add water as needed to form a thick batter.

Heat oil and spoon in batter, forming burger-sized patties. Fry until brown on one side, turn and flatten if necessary. Fry until the second side is golden too. Serve with applesauce or fruit relish.

Note: if the patties appear to flake or crumble while frying, they are too wet. Add more flour.

Fried Rice

We all eat a lot of rice, so it's nice to find a slightly different way of preparing it. The eggs and bacon in this dish add protein and make it a main dish. Fresh rice won't absorb the other flavors as well as day old, but make fresh if you must. This is a good way to use up rice from Chinese take-out.

Ingredients

Safflower oil

3 eggs

2 tablespoons minced garlic

1 teaspoon ginger

3-5 scallions, chopped

4 strips of cooked bacon

8 cups cooked rice (day old is best)

3 tablespoons thin GF tamari sauce*

In a wok or deep fry pan, bring 2 tablespoons of oil to very high heat. Add the eggs and scramble them (take care not to overcook—the eggs should be soft). Remove the eggs and coat the wok with a little more oil. Stir-fry the garlic and scallions. Add the bacon and then the rice and mix thoroughly. Add tamari then mix the eggs back in. Serve immediately.

*If you cannot find GF tamari, use Bragg's Aminos, but thin it with water or it will be too salty. If no soy is tolerated, try substituting some sesame oil. Sesame oil is very strong, however, so a teaspoon is probably enough.

Brunswick Stew

*When I first started cooking, I was armed only with the 1967 edition of **The Joy of Cooking** (a book I still consult regularly). Brunswick Chicken was one of the first things I cooked, though I'm not really sure why. There are lots of variations on this traditional stew, but the one that follows is very good and can be made on the stove or in a slow cooker.*

Ingredients

1 chicken, cut into serving pieces

1 onion, chopped coarsely

2 stalks of celery, chopped

2 cups frozen corn (substitute another vegetable if sensitive to corn)

1 cup canned butter beans, drained and rinsed (puree if your child won't eat beans)

1 1-pound can tomatoes

2 baking potatoes, peeled and cubed

2 tablespoons apple cider vinegar

1 tablespoon firmly packed brown sugar (optional)

1/3 cup GF ketchup

1 teaspoon dried marjoram

1 teaspoon dried oregano

2 tablespoons GF/CF margarine

1/2 teaspoon Tabasco

Salt and pepper (to taste)

Place chicken in a Dutch oven and add enough cold water to cover. Bring to a boil, removing any foam that forms. Add onion, celery and spices, and boil until the chicken is well cooked and nearly coming off the bones. Remove the chicken to a platter to cool.

Add the rest of the ingredients to the broth and cook for about an hour (potatoes should be fork tender).   Remove the chicken from the bones and add it back to the stew.

Socca

Here is another recipe from Lynne Davis. This makes a nice side dish. It also makes a tasty snack.

Ingredients

3 to 4 teaspoons extra virgin olive oil

1 medium onion, chopped

2 cups garbanzo bean flour (sometimes called Besan)

1 teaspoon salt

1/2 teaspoon Herbes de Provence (or Italian Seasoning)

2 cups water

Preheat oven to 350°.

Sauté the onion in a little olive oil until clear and starting to brown, and set aside. Put flour in a bowl and whisk it to remove lumps. Add salt, herbs, and water.   Mix well. Put into two oiled pie pans. Brush with a little more oil and top with cooked onions.

Bake for 30 to 35 minutes. Cut into wedges and serve as a snack or with a meal.

Pineapple Chicken

Pineapple is well tolerated by many children who are allergic to citrus, and it often makes a nice alternative. Even when following a yeast-free regimen, pineapple is acceptable (in moderation). Likewise, coconut milk is a food to which few children react.

Ingredients:

12 ounces coconut milk (use "lite" coconut milk if cutting fat)

1 pound boneless chicken breast (cut into bite sized chunks)

1 onion, chopped

1 teaspoon oil

1/4 cup uncooked rice

1/4 teaspoon ground ginger

1/2 cup canned pineapple (in juice)

1/2 teaspoon arrowroot starch

1 cup GF chicken broth

Salt and pepper to taste

Sauté onion and add chicken to the pan. Cook to brown slightly.

Add spices and rice to pan and cook, stirring constantly, for about 2 minutes. Add broth and stir to mix. Bring to a simmer, then cover and cook over low heat for 20-30 minutes (until rice absorbs liquid).

Drain pineapple well, reserving juice. Stir arrowroot into juice to make a paste. Add coconut milk to chicken, then add paste and stir until the sauce has thickened.

Curried Chicken Balls

Don't let the name fool you—this has just enough spice to be interesting. As of this writing New Morning® Crispy Rice Cereal was gluten free. Always check ingredients to be sure. These are a nice change of pace from the usual chicken nugget—use strips for "tenders" if you prefer. Great for lunch or dinner. (These can also be fried.)

Ingredients

3 cups New Morning Crispy Rice cereal, crushed to 1 1/2 cups

2 eggs*

2 tablespoons water

1/2 teaspoon curry powder

1/2 teaspoon garlic powder

1 teaspoon dried minced onion

Salt and pepper to taste

1 pound boneless chicken breast, cut into bite sized pieces

Combine eggs and water in shallow bowl or pan. Beat to combine.

In a separate shallow pan (a pie plate works well) combine cereal and spices. Dip pieces of chicken in egg, then coat with cereal mixture.

Placed coated pieces on foil covered cookie sheet and spray lightly with Pam. Bake at 375° for about 15 minutes or until chicken is tender and not pink.

*If egg intolerant, replace egg mixture with 3 tablespoon melted GF/CF margarine or ghee.

Barbequed Chicken Pie

*The original idea for this dish came from an issue of **Cooking Light** magazine, one of my favorite sources. It took a bit of fiddling to make it both comply with the diet and kid-friendly. My children both love this dish, however, and it's not too labor intensive.*

Ingredients

1 teaspoon CF margarine

Cooking spray

2 cups chopped onion

1 4.5-ounce can chopped green chilies, drained (optional)

1 small garlic clove, minced

1/4 cup cider vinegar

4 cups shredded cooked chicken breast (about 1 1/2 pounds)

2 tablespoons brown sugar

12 ounces GF bottled chili sauce

10 1/2 ounces chicken broth

One recipe Quickie-dough biscuit dough (see recipe page 216)

Preheat oven to 375°.

Melt margarine over medium-high heat in a large nonstick skillet coated with cooking spray. Add onion and garlic and sauté 5 minutes. Stir in vinegar, scraping skillet to loosen browned bits.

Add the chicken and the next 4 ingredients (chicken, brown sugar, chili sauce and broth), and cook 15 minutes or until thick, stirring occasionally. Spoon chicken mixture into 11 x 7-inch baking dish coated with cooking spray.

Make biscuit dough, roll out and cut into 11-inch strips. Place strips in a lattice fashion over chicken mixture.* Bake for 25 minutes or until lattice is golden brown; let stand 15 minutes before serving.

*If preferred, roll out dough to slightly larger circumference than your casserole dish. Place on top of chicken and trim to fit. Bake for a more traditional pie look.

Bubble and Squeak

You're more likely to find this in London than in New Jersey where I live, but this is an easy dish that makes a nice change of pace for Sunday brunch or a light supper. It is also a good way to sneak in some veggies, especially if you have a potato lover at your house. If you have other leftover veggies, dice them and toss them in too.

This is a small recipe—feel free to double it. If you don't have leftover vegetables, the parsnips and turnips can be cooked in a microwave or baked on a lightly greased cookie pan.

Ingredients

4 potatoes, peeled, cooked and cold

1 small diced onion

2 turnips, cooked and diced

2 parsnips, scraped, cooked and diced

3 strips of cooked bacon (reserve fat)

1 cup shredded Tofutti® cheese (optional)

Slice potatoes into 1/4-inch slices. Sauté onion in some bacon fat, then add potatoes to brown.

Add remaining vegetables. When almost done, stir in cheese to melt.

Macaroni and "Cheese"

Special Diets for Special Kids included a recipe for this well-loved comfort food. I offer another version here, which is slightly different—a bit more nutritious. Sesame seeds contain calcium, so while this dish might not have as much of that mineral as the real thing, it is a good substitute.

Ingredients

14 ounces GF macaroni

4 cups water

1 10-ounce pkg. soft silken tofu, drained

1 cup soymilk or DariFree

1/2 cup tahini (sesame seed paste)

1 teaspoon turmeric (optional)*

Salt

2 tablespoons dairy-free margarine or olive oil

Preheat oven to 350°. Bring water and oil to boil, then cook noodles (according to package directions) to the *al dente* stage. Drain and rinse well.

Blend tofu and "milk" in blender or food processor until smooth. Add tahini, turmeric and salt; mix until smooth.

In large bowl, stir together macaroni and "cheese" sauce. Place mixture in lightly oiled ovenproof casserole; dot with GF margarine. Bake until golden and bubbly, about 20 minutes.

*Turmeric will give the sauce the orange color of packaged macaroni and cheese, but it will change the flavor and some children may not like it. Unless your child is very sensitive to appearance (i.e., it has to "look right") you may want to omit this spice. Be warned that turmeric will stain utensils as you cook.

Nadine's Baked Ziti

Nadine Gilder is a dedicated mom who took to the GF/CF diet like a fish to water. Both she and husband Jules have created many wonderful recipes, and this is one of the best. Everyone who tastes it loves it. Through her personal consulting business, Nadine helps other parents struggling with the diet.

Ingredients:

1 pound gluten-free ziti or other noodle

1 egg, beaten

1 recipe mock ricotta*

3 cups GF/CF pasta sauce

1/4 cup chopped fresh parsley or one tablespoon of dry parsley flakes

1 teaspoon oregano

1/2 teaspoon garlic powder

1/4 teaspoon pepper

1/2 teaspoon salt

Cook the pasta in a pot of boiling water until it is al dente. Drain and rinse.

Preheat your oven to 350°.

In a large bowl, stir together 1 1/2 cups of GF/CF pasta sauce and all of the other ingredients. Spoon the pasta and sauce mixture into a 13 x 9 x 2-inch pan. Top it with 1 1/2 cups of GF/CF pasta sauce. Cover the pan with aluminum foil and bake for 30 minutes or until it is hot and bubbly.

*Nadine's original recipe calls for a 16-ounce package of firm tofu, mashed. This works very well and tastes good too.

Nadine's Outrageous Tuna (Or Chicken) Casserole

The Gilder family loves tuna casserole, so Nadine came up with a good duplicate that uses no gluten or casein. The problem is that many autism specialists are now suggesting our children eat NO FISH at all, due to the very high levels of mercury being found. Nadine's recipe will work very well with cooked chicken too, so you decide which to use. The Gilders think that the recipe is outrageously good, hence its name.

Ingredients

1 12-to-16 ounce package of GF/CF pasta

2 cans CF chunk light tuna in water (drained) or chicken

2 cans Rokeach brand mushroom soup* - Kosher for Passover (available all
　　　year round at most major supermarket chains)

1 1/2 cups frozen mixed vegetables

Cook the pasta until it is al dente, then drain and rinse with cold water. In a separate bowl, mix together the drained tuna fish, mushroom soup and mixed vegetables. Set aside while you make the white sauce.

White Sauce

4 tablespoons GF/CF margarine

4 tablespoons sweet rice flour

2 cups DariFree (already mixed with water) or other milk substitute

Preheat the oven to 350°.

Melt the margarine in a small saucepan. Add the sweet rice flour and blend (with a fork or spoon) into a paste. Add the milk substitute gradually while stirring. Stir and cook over medium heat until the sauce is smooth and thick. A thick milk such as soy or DariFree is preferred over a thin milk like rice milk.

Pour the white sauce over the fish or chicken mixture. Pour gently to distribute evenly over the pasta. Take care not to mash the pasta, and transfer the mixture to a 9 x 13-inch pan. Bake for 45 to 60 minutes until the mixture is thoroughly warmed and bubbling on top.

Optional: You can put GF/CF bread crumbs or GF/CF cornflakes on top to get a crispy topping.

*Imagine Foods also makes a good GF/CF mushroom soup. If you cannot find Rokeach brand, look for Imagine in your health food store.

Mushroom Rice

Here is another super simple way to serve rice. Brown rice will add some nutrients lacking in white rice. Omit mushrooms if following a yeast-free regimen.

Ingredients

4 cups cooked rice (brown or white)

8 ounces Imagine® mushroom soup

1/2 cup mushrooms, cleaned and sliced

1/4 cup plus one tablespoon CF margarine or ghee, melted

Preheat oven to 350°.

In a tablespoon of the margarine or ghee, sauté mushrooms and onions. Combine with rice.

In a greased casserole, alternate layers of rice and soup, ending with rice. Drizzle melted ghee on top and bake for 20 minutes or until heated through.

Taco Pie

This is a delicious and very easy main dish that most children will enjoy. It is so quick to put together that you will find yourself making it often.

Ingredients

1 pound ground beef (preferably sirloin)

1 medium onion, chopped

1 recipe taco seasoning mix (see recipe on page 224)

1 can chopped green chilis, drained

1 cup milk substitute

2 eggs

1/2 cup Quickie Baking Mix (page 216)

1/4 cup chunky salsa

Preheat oven to 400°.

Brown meat and onion over medium heat. Drain excess fat and stir in seasoning mix. Transfer meat mixture to a deep pie pan, and top with chilis and salsa.

In a separate bowl, combine milk substitute, eggs and baking mix until blended (there may be a few lumps and that's ok). Pour over meat.

Bake for about 35 minutes or until a knife inserted in the center comes out clean.

Variation: To make hamburger pie, omit the taco seasoning and salsa. Add one teaspoon salt to the meat mixture.

Easy Corned Beef and Cabbage

I'm hardly Irish, but this is great for St. Patrick's day or any day. If you think your child won't touch vegetables, puree them in the blender first.

Ingredients

1 14-ounce can vegetable or chicken broth (be sure it is GF)

2 cloves of garlic, peeled and sliced

1/2 teaspoon caraway seeds

1/4 teaspoon coarsely ground black pepper

1 small head of cabbage, cored and chopped coarsely

1 pound baby potatoes (peeling is optional)

3/4 pound thin-sliced deli corned beef*

In a deep sauté pan with lid, heat the broth, garlic, caraway seeds and pepper to boiling.

Add the cabbage and potatoes then reduce to a simmer. Cook until the potatoes are tender and remove the pan from the heat. Add the corned beef to the vegetables, and heat through.

*Be sure to read the label on the corned beef; it often contains forbidden ingredients. If possible, buy corned beef and other luncheon meats that are Kosher for Passover—they contain no corn and will usually be additive free.

Baked Tofu Teriyaki

Lynne Davis contributed several recipes to **Special Diets,** *including the wonderful Pineapple Velvet Cake. She's come through again with some delicious ideas, and this one is terrific if your child can eat soy. Lynne suggests starting this one the night before so the tofu has a long time to marinate. I like serving this with rice.*

Ingredients

2 packages (12.3 ounce) extra firm lite tofu

6 tablespoons Bragg Liquid Aminos

Juice of one small lemon

2 tablespoons sesame oil

3 tablespoons honey

3 cloves garlic, minced

2 teaspoons minced gingerroot

3 green onions, minced

1/2 teaspoon freshly ground black pepper

Put the tofu in a colander, and place a plate on top of it. Then add some weight to press out the excess water (a one-pound bag of dried beans works nicely). Put the colander over a bowl and refrigerate it for 30 minutes. Mix the remaining ingredients in a small bowl to make the marinade.

Cut the pressed tofu into cubes. Coat the bottom of an oven-proof glass dish with some of the marinade. You don't want to crowd the tofu so use two dishes if necessary. Add the tofu, separating the cubes. Pour the marinade over the cubes. Spoon it up and over the cubes until they are well coated.

Refrigerate the tofu for at least 6 hours, or even overnight. Turn the cubes several times if you think of it. Do not drain the marinade. Bake the tofu for 45 minutes at 350°.

Baked Hush Puppies

Serve these tasty little gems instead of bread or crackers when you're having chili or other soups. The fact that they are baked means they are reasonably healthful, but you could fry them if you prefer extra crispy pups. If corn is not tolerated, use a cream-of-rice-style hot cereal (not instant).

Ingredients

1/2 cup Gift of Nature® Flour mixture

1/2 cup yellow cornmeal

2 cups New Morning Crispy Rice cereal, crushed

1 teaspoon sugar (optional)

2 teaspoons baking powder

1/2 teaspoon salt

1/8 teaspoon red pepper

2 teaspoons xanthan gum

2 eggs

2 tablespoons oil

1/2 cup milk substitute

1/2 teaspoon garlic

Cooking spray

Preheat oven to 425°.

In medium bowl, stir together flour, cornmeal, cereal and other dry ingredients. Set aside. In large bowl beat together eggs, milk substitute and oil until well mixed. Stir in garlic. Add to flour mixture, mixing until well combined.

Use hands to form little balls and portion into 24 mini-muffin pan cups coated with spray.

Bake for 15-20 minutes or until light brown.

Buffalo Wings

My kids love wings. They are easy to make, either baked in the oven or on the grill. The important thing is the marinade. Be sure to let them marinate overnight if possible. The spiciness can be adjusted to your taste, of course. Though traditionally served with blue cheese dressing, try the Ranch dressing recipe on page 220. Most recipes call for frying, but I like to grill or bake them.

Ingredients

4 pounds chicken wings

1 cup apple cider vinegar

2 tablespoons oil

2 tablespoons GF Worcestershire sauce*

1 teaspoon garlic powder

1 teaspoon chili powder

1 teaspoon salt

Tabasco to taste (2-3 teaspoons for mild wings, 1 tablespoon or more for really spicy wings).

Marinate in a casserole dish or in a large, strong plastic bag (a bag has the advantage that you can mix the wings around every few hours without having to unwrap them). If using a dish, be sure to cover tightly but unwrap and stir the wings around.

Bake at 400° for 30-40 minutes or until done, or grill.

If grilling, use the marinade to brush the wings as they cook. If baking, add marinade as needed to prevent burning and sticking.

*As of this writing, Lea & Perrins Worcestershire is GF.

Hungarian Goulash

There is a big difference between imported sweet paprika and the domestic stuff, which really just makes food red. Be sure to buy the real thing when making goulash. This recipe uses beef chuck, but you can upgrade to a nicer cut of beef or veal cubes if you prefer. Delicious served with noodles and, if soy is tolerated, mock sour cream. Often it is served with dumplings instead (see recipe for dumplings on page 215).

Ingredients

2 pounds beef chuck, cubed

2 onions, chopped

2 tablespoons shortening

2 tablespoons imported sweet paprika

1 bay leaf

4 cups water

4 potatoes, peeled and diced

1/4 teaspoon black pepper

Salt to taste

Cut meat into 1-inch cubes and add approximately 1/2 teaspoon salt. Brown meat in shortening, then add onions and paprika. Let meat simmer in its own juice along with salt and paprika for about an hour on low heat. Add water, diced potatoes and remaining salt. Cover and simmer until potatoes are done and meat is tender.

Hungarian Chicken

This recipe is not, I fear, authentic Hungarian. It is good, however, and it is quite easy to prepare.

Ingredients

1 chicken, cut into serving pieces

1 15-ounce can stewed tomatoes

1 onion, diced

2 tablespoons sweet paprika

1 teaspoon chili powder

1 clove garlic or one teaspoon garlic powder

2 tablespoons chili sauce

1/2 teaspoon dried basic

1/2 teaspoon dried parsley

1 tablespoon GF/CF margarine or olive oil

Preheat oven to 375°.

Brown chicken on a baking sheet for about 40 minutes. Lower oven temperature to 350°.

In a saucepan, sauté onion in oil or margarine. When onions are soft, add other ingredients and cook for a few minutes over medium heat. Place the chicken in an ovenproof casserole, cover with sauce and then bake for 45-60 minutes.

Schnitzel

Weiner schnitzel is typically made with veal, but pork tenderloin makes a really good and simple dish. I only recently discovered pork tenderloin, when it was on special at my store. We all liked it so much that I buy it frequently now. It is easy to prepare and very versatile. You can certainly use veal if you prefer.

Ingredients

1 pork tenderloin, about one pound

1 egg

1 cup GF/CF bread crumbs (I prefer Dr. Schaar's®, available from Glutino)

2 tablespoons oil

1/2 teaspoon salt

1/2 teaspoon pepper

1/2 teaspoon garlic powder

Cut the pork tenderloin crosswise into approximately 8 slices. Place each slice between 2 sheets of plastic wrap and gently pound pork with a rolling pin until about 1/4 inch thick.

Place the egg in a shallow bowl and beat. Place the breadcrumbs in pie pans and season with the salt, pepper and garlic powder.

Heat oil in large skillet over medium-high heat until hot.

Dip each pork piece in egg and then dip in breadcrumbs to coat. Place coated pork slices into hot oil and cook about 3 minutes on each side, until golden.

Serve with GF noodles.

Pork Stew

When I began working at home, I had more time to spend shopping, and often explored new neighborhoods and stores. In one I found many exotic root vegetables. After doing a bit of research, I realized that these roots, while exotic to me, are everyday fare in many Latino communities. They are inexpensive and are a nice change from potatoes. They are also great for people rotating foods.

Ingredients

$2^1/2$ pounds assorted Latin roots (including malanga, yucca, boniato and true yam)

2 tablespoons safflower oil

1 pound boneless pork loin trimmed of fat and cut into half-inch cubes

Salt and freshly ground black pepper to taste

1 onion, diced

2 tablespoons garlic, minced

1 tablespoon paprika

1 teaspoon red or green chili, minced

2 teaspoons ground cumin

2 quarts chicken stock

Juice of one lime

Peel roots and tubers (if using yucca or true yams, take care to peel off the bitter under layer). Dice and set aside in a large bowl. Fill with water to cover.

Heat oil over medium-high heat in a large pan. Sprinkle pork with salt and pepper; add to the pan and brown on all sides, 5 to 7 minutes. Remove and set aside.

Drain all but one tablespoon of fat from the pan, add the onion, and sauté over medium heat, stirring occasionally. Cook until translucent, about 5 to 7 minutes. Add garlic, paprika, chilies and cumin, and sauté one minute more.

Add stock and reserved root vegetables, and bring just to a boil. Reduce heat to very low, and simmer, stirring occasionally, for about 30 minutes or until pork is tender and roots are easily pierced with a fork. Stir in the lime juice.

Veal Stew

My friend Annie gave me this recipe years ago. It came from her mother, Judith Williams, and it is delicious. If soy is not tolerated you can omit the mock sour cream. Though it will be a much different dish, it will still be good. Don't forget that the alcohol in the wine will cook out of the final product.

Ingredients

3 pounds veal

1 1/2 cups Tofutti Sour Supreme®

1 large onion, chopped

1/4 - 1/2 cup white wine

1/2 cup mushrooms, chopped

3 tablespoons imported sweet paprika

Oil

Sauté onions in oil, then stir in veal. Brown the meat on all sides, then add all ingredients except Sour Supreme.

Cover and cook over low heat until the meat is tender. Add Sour Supreme when meat is fully cooked, and cook gently until heated through. Serve with GF noodles.

Stir-fried Pork

Here's another way to use pork tenderloin. It's tasty and you can use it to slip in some veggies. If you're lucky, your kids won't even notice.

Ingredients:

Cooking spray

4 cups onion, sliced vertically

1 cup broccoli florets, chopped very fine

1 pork tenderloin, cut into thin slices

1/2 cup chopped green onions

1 tablespoon sugar (optional)

1 tablespoon fresh ginger, peeled and minced.

3 garlic cloves, minced

1/2 cup chicken broth

3 tablespoons GF soy or tamari sauce

1/2 cup chopped dry-roasted cashews or almonds

2 teaspoons sesame oil

2 cups hot cooked long-grain rice

Place a large nonstick skillet coated with cooking spray over medium-high heat.

Add onion; cook 8 minutes, stirring occasionally. Remove the onion from pan and place in a bowl.

Recoat pan with cooking spray. Add broccoli; stir-fry 3 minutes. Add broccoli to onion.

Recoat pan with cooking spray. Add pork and red pepper; stir-fry 4 minutes or until pork loses its pink color.

Reduce heat. Stir in the green onions, sugar, ginger, and garlic, and cook 30 seconds, stirring constantly.

Stir in onion mixture, chicken broth, soy sauce, and cashews; cook 1 minute. Drizzle with sesame oil. Serve with rice.

Mom's Cassoulet

Ok, so Mom isn't really French, and this isn't a truly authentic cassoulet. The real thing calls for all kinds of fancy (and expensive) ingredients, and takes days to cook.

But this recipe is delicious and fairly easy and makes a wonderful meal on a cold winter day. Try it—it has so many different things in it that everyone will find something they like, even if it means picking a little.

Mom says, "Try it, it's worth the trouble."

If you prefer, cook the beans the day before and refrigerate them until you are ready to prepare the dish.

Ingredients

1 pound lean lamb chunks

1/2 pound sausage, cut into chunks

2 cloves of garlic

2 onions, sliced

1 pound chicken, boned and skinned and cut into chunks

1/2 pound white beans

2 cups red wine

1-3 sprigs of parsley

1 bay leaf

Salt and pepper to taste

Olive or safflower oil (for sautéing)

Brown lamb in a little olive or safflower oil. Remove lamb and brown the chicken, then remove the chicken and brown the sausage.

Brown onions and garlic in the same pan over low heat. Cook until very dark and set aside.

Cook the beans according to the package directions, but cook them until they are almost, but not completely, done.

In a very large casserole, layer lamb, sausage, chicken, onions and beans. Pour wine over it all. Sprinkle top with chopped parsley and toss in your bay leaf.

Cover tightly and bake for about 4 hours in a slow oven (250°). Most of the liquid should be gone and the meats and beans will be soft.

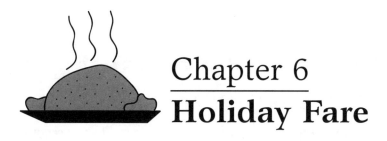

Chapter 6
Holiday Fare

*T*he holiday season—can you remember how exciting it was when you were a child? Filled with special events and treats that happen just once a year, most kids count the minutes as the holidays draw near.

For families with special needs children, however, the season is very different. All the elements that make the season so exciting for typical kids seem to bring out the very worst in autistic spectrum children.

When you rely on predictability to make sense of your world, all the changes in your routine conspire to make this special time of year a disaster. Behaviors you haven't seen in months may reappear, and your blood pressure may rise as the temperatures fall. Instead of eager anticipation, you may find yourself filled with dread as the holidays approach.

Even without a special needs child, the holidays can be trying. Anyone who cooks for his or her family knows how stressful holidays can be. Making plans, shopping and scheduling oven time can cause major headaches. Now add to all this the need to order ahead from specialty food companies and make extra trips to health food stores—is it any wonder that the season seems more trying than joyful?

If ever there is a time when we want to fall back on old eating habits, this is it. Parents may decide to forego the gluten and casein-free diet because adding **special** foods to an already full menu is too hard or too expensive. Sometimes parents fear that their child will be missing something wonderful, or perhaps they can't find good recipes that will make the meal festive.

Tempting as this might be, holidays are definitely not the time to ease up on dietary restrictions. With the stress inherent in the season, why add to it with behavioral regressions made worse by dietary infractions? Instead, plan ahead and you can hold your resolve and maintain the diet during the holidays, all without sacrificing good food and special treats.

The recipes in this chapter should make it easy to hold your resolve during the holidays. I believe that if you make the GF/CF specialties good enough, you can make them instead of your old recipes rather than adding more to the table.

Most of the recipes that follow were created with the BIG holidays in mind (Christmas and Thanksgiving), but there are others included that would be appropriate for other holidays.

Most families roast a bird for Thanksgiving and Christmas. As long as you avoid birds that have been injected with flavorings, you won't need a special recipe to make a gluten and casein-free turkey or goose. Let's be honest though—the bird may just be an excuse to eat stuffing and gravy. These are a little trickier to make gluten free, but never fear, it can be done.

Gravy

There's no mystery to making gluten-free gravy. While the turkey is roasting, add 6 cups of chicken stock to a saucepan, bring to a boil, then cook the giblets and neck. Lower the heat and let simmer for about an hour (it should reduce to 4 cups). Add 2-4 tablespoons of the roasting pan fat to the mixture and cook on high heat until reduced to 2 cups. Remove the giblets and neck, and pour 1/2 cup of the liquid into a small bowl. Add 3 tablespoons of cornstarch to the 1/2 cup of liquid and stir until well dissolved. Add the liquid back to the pan and cook over low heat, stirring often, until the gravy has thickened.

If your child cannot eat corn products, sweet rice flour or tapioca starch may be substituted.

Cranberry Sauce Deluxe

I love cranberry sauce and make it often. I generally use the recipe on the back of the Ocean Spray® package, which is easy to make and very good. I often add other ingredients, usually dried cherries. Recently my mother suggested the following additions to the cranberries. Please note that cranberries are very sour, so recipes call for lots of sugar. I have found that several of the substitute sweeteners work very well (e.g., xylitol or Sucralose®).

As cranberry sauce cooks, add any or all of the following:

5-6 finely cut dried apricots

6 prunes, chopped

3 dried peaches, chopped

1/2 cup dried cherries

Roast Goose

Just about everyone has roasted a turkey for a holiday meal. Geese and ducks are less commonly served, even though they are tasty and easy to make.

Geese, like all water fowl, need a lot of fat to keep warm. This means they are very delicious, but it also means that you don't get a whole lot of flesh from even a large bird. In fact, by the time the fat has melted away, you probably need to allow for a pound per person. Really large geese aren't that easy to find, so you may need to buy more than one small bird if you are feeding a crowd of more than eight. You can use any stuffing you would use for turkey, or you can skip it altogether.

Ingredients

1 8-lb goose

Salt

Pepper

12 slices of bacon

2 tablespoons GF breadcrumbs

1/4 cup fresh herbs, minced (e.g. parsley, basil, thyme)

1 tablespoon Dijon mustard

Preheat the oven to 425°.

Remove giblets and set aside for making stuffing desired (see recipes for GF Stuffing page 130). Pierce the skin of the bird with a fork.

If you stuff the bird, fill the body and neck cavity with stuffing. If you choose not to stuff the goose, place a large orange in the body cavity.

Place the bird on a meat rack in a roasting pan. Cover the bird with bacon and roast for 45 minutes, pouring off fat as needed. Reduce oven heat to 375° and bake for another 60 to 90 minutes (longer if the bird is stuffed).

Chop the bacon very finely and mix with herbs and GF breadcrumbs. Spread mustard on goose and cover with breadcrumbs and bake another 20-30 minutes, or until the meat is tender and the juice runs clear.

Root-Vegetable Mashed Potatoes With Chestnuts

This dish makes a very nice change of pace from plain mashed potatoes. The parsnips are tolerated even by very food sensitive children, and they add some extra nutrients and fiber. Chestnuts are also well tolerated, and are the only nut that is truly low in fat.

Ingredients

4 cups potatoes, peeled and cubed (Yukon gold potatoes work very well)

2 cups parsnips, peeled and sliced

5 garlic cloves, peeled

1/4 cup fresh parsley, chopped

1/4 cup GF chicken broth

1 tablespoon CF margarine

1/2 cup chestnuts, cooked, shelled and chopped

Salt and pepper to taste

Place the potatoes, parsnips and garlic in a large saucepan. Cover with water and bring to a boil. Cook the vegetables for 20 minutes or until very tender. Drain. Return the potato mixture to the pan, add broth, margarine and parsley. Using a hand mixer set at medium speed, beat until smooth. Stir in chestnuts.

GF Bread Stuffing

Everyone has a favorite turkey stuffing recipe. Last Thanksgiving I used one that appeared in the Miss Robens catalogue, and modified it a little to suit my family's taste. I found that using GF English Muffins worked especially well, because they are thick enough to cut into cubes. I used the muffins made by Foods By George®, a GF bakery here in New Jersey. Others would work too, as would GF bread.

According to my mother, a loose rule of thumb says about 10 cups of bread pieces makes enough for a 10-pound bird.

Ingredients

5-6 Cups GF English Muffins, buns or bread, cut into 2" pieces

2 tablespoons oil

3 cups chopped celery

2 cups chopped onion

1 teaspoon salt

1 teaspoon thyme

1 teaspoon parsley

Black pepper

1 1/2 cups GF broth

Preheat oven to 400°

Cut bread or muffins into 2" cubes and spread on a cookie sheet. Toast in a slow oven (325° or lower) for 30 minutes or so. Shake the pan or turn with a spatula every 10 minutes. The cubes should be well dried. They do not need to be browned but it is fine if they are.

Sauté chopped celery and onions in oil over medium heat until soft. Add spices and pepper. Pour in chicken stock and simmer over low heat for 15 to 20 minutes.

Add the bread to the saucepan, and combine until the bread is fully saturated in sauce and seasonings. Transfer to a covered casserole dish and bake for 40-50 minutes.

Mashed Sweet Potatoes

Sweet potatoes don't have to be made dessert-sweet. Mash them instead of regular russet potatoes for a nice holiday starch.

Ingredients

4 sweet potatoes, baked and peeled

6 tablespoons CF margarine

1/2 cup Darifree or soy milk, warmed

1 egg, lightly beaten

1/2 teaspoon nutmeg (optional)

Salt and pepper to taste

Preheat oven to 350°

In a large bowl, mash roasted sweet potatoes with margarine. Beat in milk substitute, egg and nutmeg. Transfer to a lightly greased casserole and bake for 25 minutes. Serve hot.

Mom's Bread Stuffing

This is a GF version of my mother's bread stuffing, a tradition at her table. While it is a delicious stuffing, it does call for eggs and so will not be suitable for everyone.

Mom has passed her dislike of the herb sage down to me, so like Mom, I have omitted it from any stuffing I make. If you like sage, however, go ahead and add a teaspoon of it. I don't know that I have ever seen a stuffing recipe that did not call for it.

Mom's instructions were a bit, well, loose. I've tried to standardize measurements, but you may want to tinker a bit.

Ingredients

1 loaf of 2-day-old ANDI Wunderbread*

1 quart GF chicken broth

3 tablespoons GF/CF margarine, or ghee

2 onions, chopped

3 stalks of celery, chopped

2 cups mushrooms, cleaned and sliced

2 eggs, beaten

Giblets from bird being cooked

Tear or cut bread into small chunks and place in large mixing bowl. Set aside.

Place giblets in a pot and cover with chicken broth (add water if necessary). Add one onion, salt and pepper to taste. Bring to a boil and simmer slowly until giblets are tender. Don't let the liquid boil out—add water if necessary. Set aside.

In a fry pan, sauté finely diced celery, the second onion and mushrooms until lightly browned. If desired, chop up giblets into small pieces and add to the fried onion mixture. (If preferred, leave them out.)

Pour 2 to 3 cups of the giblet broth over the torn bread. It should be very moist. Add the eggs and sautéed onion mix. Mix well.

Here's where you have to use your own judgment, because, according to Mom, you want it quite moist, but not too moist. It shouldn't be "running" wet. If you accidentally get it too wet, add more bread. Add salt and pepper and whatever herbs your family enjoys.

If you bake the stuffing out of the bird, it will take approximately 35-40 minutes at 350°.

*ANDI Wunderbread mix can be purchased from Miss Roben's. Or bake your own, following the recipe for Marci's bread in **Special Diets for Special Kids** (page 140). If you prefer, use GF English Muffins as described for GF Bread Stuffing.

Rice Stuffing

There's no law that says stuffing must be made from bread. Rice stuffing makes a delicious change of pace, and since it can be baked in a casserole there really is no reason to make it only when serving a large holiday meal. Wild rice has a nutty flavor and a great texture. If your family doesn't like a "soggy" bread type stuffing, give this a try.

Ingredients

1/2 cup onion, chopped

1/2 cup celery, chopped

1/4 cup CF margarine (may substitute coconut butter or ghee)

1/2 cup wild rice, rinsed and drained

4 cups GF chicken stock

1 cup long grain rice (I like Basmati rice, an aromatic Indian rice)

3 cups Yukon Gold potatoes, peeled and chopped

1/2 teaspoon salt

1/2 teaspoon pepper

1/2 cup pecans, chopped

1/2 cup fresh parsley or one tablespoon dried parsley

Preheat oven to 325°.

In a large saucepan, sauté onion and celery in margarine until soft. Add wild rice and broth and bring to a boil. Reduce heat, cover and simmer 20 minutes.

Add white rice, potatoes and seasonings, and return to the boil. Reduce heat and simmer, covered, for 20 minutes or until the rice is cooked and the liquid has been absorbed. Add parsley and nuts and bake in a lightly greased 2-quart casserole for 50 minutes.

Cranberry Nut Stuffing

I adore cranberries. Every November, when they first make their appearance in the grocery store, I buy enough to last the year. They freeze very well, and I love to throw them into applesauce and other dishes. I also really like dried cranberries, which used to be hard to find but now are widely available. This recipe uses dried cranberries and nuts, and is a really nice change of pace.

Ingredients

1/2 cup celery, chopped

1/2 cup onion, chopped

1/4 cup CF margarine

1/2 teaspoon dried thyme

1/2 teaspoon dried marjoram

6 cups bread (preferably GF English Muffins), cubed and toasted lightly

1/2 cup dried cranberries

1/2 cup chopped nuts (preferably pecans or hazelnuts)

1/2 cup GF chicken broth

Preheat oven to 325°.

Sauté celery and onions in margarine and remove from heat when tender. Add herbs, salt, pepper to taste.

Place bread cubes in a mixing bowl and add celery mixture and cranberries. Use enough broth to moisten well.

Bake in a covered casserole for 30 to 45 minutes.

Sweet Noodle Kugel

This recipe works well with rice noodles—use the broadest noodle you can find (probably a fettuccini) and break into short pieces before boiling. I find that Tinkayada® noodles work well with this recipe. Sweet kugel is often served at holiday meals in Jewish homes; it is a side dish rather than a dessert.

Ingredients

1 pound rice noodles, cooked & drained

6 eggs

1 cup apricot jam

1 cup white raisins or dried apricot bits

2 teaspoons salt

1 teaspoon cinnamon

2 teaspoons vanilla

1/2 cup GF/CF margarine, melted

4 tablespoons sugar

1 teaspoon sugar

In a large bowl, beat the eggs well. Add jam, raisins, salt, cinnamon and vanilla. Mix thoroughly. Stir in noodles. If mixture seems dry, add up to 1/2 cup water.

Pour into a 9 x 13-inch pan, greased. Pour melted margarine on top and sprinkle with cinnamon and sugar mixture. Bake at 375° for 45 minutes. Serve warm or at room temperature.

Stuffed Pork Tenderloin

This recipe is delicious and is deceptively easy (i.e., it will look as though you really fussed). If you are not feeding a large crowd, this can make a very nice main course. Any stuffing recipe would work with this recipe.

As usual, I have omitted the sage but if you like it, use $1/2$ teaspoon.

Cube the English muffins and leave them out to dry for a day. If you don't remember to do this, just put them on a cookie sheet and toast in a 325° oven for 30 minutes or so, until well dried out. If you have leftover stuffing, skip right to slicing the meat and stuffing.

Ingredients

1 $1/2$ pound pork tenderloin

$1/2$ cup chopped onion

$1/2$ cup chopped celery

1 $1/2$ cups chicken broth

6 cups GF English Muffins, cubed and dry

$1/2$ teaspoon dried thyme

1 teaspoon dried marjoram

1 teaspoon dried parsley

$1/2$ teaspoon salt

1 teaspoon pepper

Preheat oven to 350°.

In a large saucepan, combine onion, celery and broth. Simmer, covered, on low until vegetables are soft. Add bread and herbs and mix until blended. Set aside.

Slice pork into $1/4$-inch slices. Arrange half of the slices in a baking pan that has been sprayed with non-stick cooking spray. Top with the stuffing. Place remaining pork slices on stuffing. Sprinkle with remaining seasonings. Cover with aluminum foil. Bake for 30 minutes or until pork is no longer pink.

Roast Leg of Lamb

If your family likes lamb, roasting a leg of lamb is another great choice of the holidays. My husband's family is French, and it was at my mother-in-law's table that I first had a fabulous "gigot" smothered in garlic and cooked deliciously rare. Served with small potatoes or just about anything you want, this will be a wonderful centerpiece for your meal and won't cost you hours of hard labor in the kitchen.

Ingredients

6-pound leg of lamb, bone in

1/4 cup Dijon mustard

2 tablespoons lemon juice

4 cloves fresh garlic, mince

1 tablespoon fresh rosemary, finely chopped

1 tablespoon fresh thyme, finely chopped

2 tablespoons extra virgin olive oil

1 large onion, peeled and chopped

1 tablespoon fresh mint, finely chopped

Kosher or coarse salt

Pepper to taste

Preheat oven to 350°.

Trim excess fat from the lamb, and season with salt and pepper. Combine the mustard, lemon juice, garlic and herbs in a blender. Blend to emulsify. Slowly trickle in the olive oil.

At least an hour before roasting, baste the lamb with the mustard mixture, and set it on a rack in a heavy-duty roasting pan.

Roast the lamb for 1 to 1 1/4 hours for medium rare (140°-145° on meat ther-mometer). Roast for 1 1/4 to 1 1/2 hours for well-done meat (160°-165° on meat thermometer).

Remove the lamb from the roasting pan and place on a warm platter. Let the lamb rest for 15 minutes before carving.

Pour off pan drippings and remove as much fat as possible. Season to taste and serve with the meat.

Basic Pork Tenderloin

Even when your holidays are GF/CF, you do have choices beyond roasting a bird. Most people know how to bake a ham or prepare a roast beef, but I think that pork tenderloin can be delicious and very festive. I only recently discovered the joys of pork tenderloin, and have prepared it several different ways.

Ingredients

3-pound pork tenderloin

2 tart, firm-fleshed pears

2 cups onion, chopped

3 cloves of garlic, peeled and chopped

3 tablespoons olive oil

3/4 cup chicken broth

2 tablespoons apple cider vinegar

1 teaspoon prepared mustard

Preheat oven to 425°.

Brown the meat in a large pan and remove to a platter. In the same pan sauté the onions and garlic for 5 minutes. Add the pears and cook for 2 minutes more. Add broth, vinegar and mustard and stir well. Add salt and pepper to taste.

Place pork in a baking pan and cover with the cooked mixture. Cover with foil and bake for 30 minutes to 1 hour—meat thermometer should read 170° for fully cooked pork. Let rest for 10 minutes before slicing. Serve with the gravy and potatoes or rice.

Yam Casserole

*I didn't learn to like yams until I was an adult, but at last Thanksgiving's dinner even the children liked them. For some reason people want a really sweet potato dish for Thanksgiving, and this is a tasty one. A recipe in the on-line version of **Cooking Light Magazine** inspired this dish. It is very sweet—almost like a dessert.*

Ingredients

3 $1/2$ pounds yams or sweet potatoes

5 tablespoons CF margarine, melted

3 eggs, beaten

$1/2$ cup Darifree or soy milk

1 cup dark brown sugar

4 tablespoons CF margarine, softened

4 tablespoons GF flour

1 cup coarsely chopped pecans

$1/4$ teaspoon each of salt, cinnamon and nutmeg

$1/2$ teaspoon vanilla

Preheat oven to 350°.

Bake yams until tender when pierced, about 1 to 1 $1/2$ hours. Remove from oven and let cool. Increase oven temperature to 375°.

Scoop out the pulp from the yams. Place in a large bowl and mash until smooth. You should have 4 cups. Whisk melted margarine and eggs into yams. In a small saucepan heat the Darifree, then stir the Darifree, along with $1/2$ cup of the sugar, into the yams. Blend thoroughly. Spread the mixture into a greased 11 x 17-inch baking dish. Mix the remaining $1/2$ cup sugar, softened margarine and flour until crumbly. Stir in the remaining ingredients. Sprinkle over the yam casserole. Bake until topping is crusty, about 30 minutes.

Vegetarian Kishke

An Internet acquaintance, Aviva Mandl, sent me this recipe last Passover.

"Kishke" is the Yiddish word for intestines, and it is definitely not a vegetarian dish. However, this version of mock kishke contains no meat of any kind. It is a delicious recipe and is very easy to make. It would be a good side dish for any holiday meal, and is a simple way to slip some veggies into your kids. Potato pancake (latke) mix is available year round.

If you double the recipe, form the rolls and freeze them before baking. Later, you can bake them without thawing but you will need to add 15-20 minutes more baking time.

Ingredients

2 carrots, cleaned and sliced

2 stalks of celery, chopped

1 small or medium onion, peeled and chopped

2 eggs

1/4 cup of oil

1 6-ounce box of Potato Pancake Mix

Preheat oven to 350°.

Grind onion, carrots and celery in a food processor.   Put into a large mixing bowl. Add the box of potato pancake mix, eggs and oil.   Mix well and spoon onto 2 lengths of foil to form two rolls, approximately 2 inches in diameter by 8 inches long. Wrap and pinch the ends of each.

Bake at 350° for one hour.   Remove from the oven and let stand about 10 minutes.   Unwrap foil and slice into pieces to serve.

Roasted Vegetables

When the holiday table is groaning with heavy dishes and lots of artery clogging goodies, it is nice to include something light and virtuous.

A few years ago my mother started serving roasted veggies with her holiday meals, and I've taken a page from her book. Even if your kids aren't big veggie eaters, they will probably accept the potatoes. Adjust the amounts to the number of people at your table, and don't save these just for holidays.

You can also make these on the grill for a great addition to any picnic.

Ingredients

Potatoes (one or more varieties)

Parsnips

Sweet potatoes

Carrots

Onions

Any other root vegetable

Cut all the vegetables into large chunks. Spread them out on a cookie sheet that has been lightly sprayed with cooking oil. Drizzle with olive or other oil, and season with salt and pepper.

Roast at 425° for 40 minutes. Turn oven down to 375° and roast for another 20 minutes.

Serve hot or just warm.

Orange Sweet Potatoes with Gingersnap Topping

*Lesley Roubinek and her husband Al run Kitchen Collectibles, a company that makes and sells copper cookie cutters and all kinds of specialty ingredients and equipment associated with cookie making. I found Kitchen Collectibles while searching the Internet for a cookie cutter shaped like New Jersey, and was amazed that their address was directly across the street from my father's office in Omaha, Nebraska. They make and sell wonderful products, and Lesley writes an electronic newsletter that goes out to thousands of cookie bakers every week. Around the holidays she posted the following recipe, which I have modified slightly. Check out their website at **www.kitchengifts.com** if you like to bake. You can join her list from the website.*

Ingredients

7 large sweet potatoes (about 5 pounds)

1/4 cup CF margarine, softened

1/4 cup brown sugar, firmly packed

1/4 cup unsweetened pineapple juice

1/4 cup orange marmalade

1 tablespoon fresh, finely grated, peeled gingerroot

2 teaspoons salt

For topping:

14 3-inch, crisp GF gingersnaps, broken into pieces (about 3 cups)

6 tablespoons CF margarine, cut into pieces

Preheat oven to 450° F. and grease a 13 x 9 x 2-inch baking dish,.

Prick potatoes and bake on a foil-lined baking sheet in middle of oven until very soft, about 1 1/2 hours.

Scoop flesh into a large bowl and mash with margarine, sugar, juice, marmalade, gingerroot, and salt. Spread potato mixture evenly in baking dish. Potato mixture may be made a day ahead and chilled, covered. Bring potato mixture to room temperature before proceeding.

In a food processor grind cookies fine. Add margarine and pulse motor until mixture resembles soft cookie dough. Wrap topping in wax paper and chill until firm, about 2 hours. Topping may be made a day ahead and chilled, covered.

Preheat oven to 400°F. Crumble topping over potato mixture and bake in middle of oven until topping is browned lightly, about 25 minutes.

Dairy-Free Pumpkin Pie

*Karyn Seroussi modified a recipe she found in a magazine, and I modified it even further. The result was a pumpkin pie that I would put up against any dairy-filled pie. I included a few recipes for crusts in **Special Diets** but face it, who has time during the holidays? Plan ahead and buy a good piecrust mix from Miss Robens or the Gluten Free Pantry and spend your time on the rest of the meal.*

Ingredients

1 15-ounce can pumpkin

12.5 ounces firm tofu

1/2 cup sugar

1/4 cup brown sugar

1 tablespoon molasses

2 eggs

1 1/2 teaspoons ground cinnamon

3/4 teaspoon ground ginger

1/4 teaspoon ground nutmeg

1/4 teaspoon ground cloves

Preheat oven to 350°.

Combine all ingredients in blender or food processor and mix until smooth. Mixture should be very thick, like whipped cream, but not as stiff as mashed potatoes.

Pour into an unbaked 9" piecrust. Pour any excess into greased custard cups. Bake for 60-65 minutes in center of oven, until crust is golden brown and center looks firm. Cool before serving.

You may be asking how you can serve a pumpkin pie without whipped cream. Good question. If your child tolerates corn products, then finding a good substitute is easy. Because people who keep kosher do not mix dairy with meat products, there are many products that are specifically formulated to be used with either. These are called *Pareue,* or sometimes *Parve.* If you cannot find it near you, you can order it from **www.mykoshermarket.com.** You can also try **www.kosher.com.** Note: both close several days before Passover, so shop early.

There are several brands available, including one called Rich's Rich Whip. These products are quite heavily sweetened with corn syrup, and contain more preservatives than I would normally feel comfortable recommending. But we're talking about a special treat, for a special occasion, so it's your call.

If your child cannot tolerate corn but can eat nuts and soy, visit your health food store and look for Now And Zen's "Hip Whip®." Packaged in a tub like Cool Whip, it contains water, grape juice concentrate, expeller pressed high oleic canola oil, cocoa butter, tofu, brown rice syrup, cashew butter and pure vanilla extract. It does not taste as much like whipped cream as the kosher products, but it may be a good choice for some families.

Meringue Turkeys

No, I haven't lost it here. Once in a while though, inspiration is born of desperation.

Last Thanksgiving I invited over another family whose son has many food allergies, in addition to being gluten and casein free. I had made some meringue to top a pie and had not used it all. I lined a baking sheet with parchment, added a tiny bit of pink food coloring (natural, from Dancing Deer, Inc.) to a small portion of the meringue, some cocoa to another spoonful and quickly fashioned some turkey cookies. They were a huge hit with all the kids.

If you are not experienced with a pastry bag, practice these ahead of time—you can eat the misshapen birds. If you have silpat baking mats, they are perfect for meringues. If not, be sure to line the pan with parchment.   Do NOT grease the pans.

Ingredients

8 egg whites (about 1 cup)

2 cups sugar

1/2 teaspoon cream of tartar (or use meringue powder, which already

   contains sugar)

1/2 cup GF/CF chocolate chips, melted

Preheat oven to 250°.

Beat the egg white until foamy, and then add cream of tartar. Continue beating, adding the sugar very gradually. Beat mixture until fluffy and stiff (but not dry.)

Divide meringue into three bowls and tint one with the color of your choice, one with cocoa and leave the third plain.

Fill a pastry bag (I always use disposable bags) with the cocoa meringue. Using a round tip (e.g., number 4) pipe fan-shaped cookies until you have used all the meringue.

Rinse out the pastry tip and put it in a clean pastry bag. Fill the second bag with the plain meringue. Starting near the bottom of your "fan," place the pastry tip on the cookie and squeeze out some meringue as you bring the tip up and over, forming an "s" shape. You are creating the neck and head of your turkey. Drag out the tip as you finish the head, and your turkey's face will have a pointy end. It doesn't have to be perfect. If you prefer, you can pipe the neck-head "s" as a separate cookie, and attach it after baking with melted chocolate.

Use the colored meringue in yet another bag to color the edges of the fan (which are now the feathers of the turkey). Use melted chocolate to make "eyes".

Bake for about a half hour, or until the turkeys are dry but not brown. Turn the oven off and let them sit until the oven is completely cool.

If you make meringues ahead of time, store them in a perfectly airtight container or they will not be crispy. Don't even attempt this if the humidity is high— meringues and humid or rainy days do not mix. You will create a sticky mess and a lot of frustration.

Cut-Out Cookies

It is traditional in most families to make cutout cookies for Christmas. This recipe will make a tasty (and not too sweet) dough that can stand up to your rolling pin.   Be sure to use decorative items that are gluten free—most sprinkles contain wheat.

Ingredients

3/4 cup CF margarine

3/4 cup sugar

2 eggs

2 teaspoons GF vanilla

1/4 teaspoon salt

2 cups GF flour mix*

2 teaspoons xanthan gum

1/4 teaspoon baking soda

1/4 teaspoon baking powder

Preheat oven to 350°.

In large bowl, cream margarine and sugar. Beat in eggs and vanilla until smooth.

Combine dry ingredients in a separate bowl and then add them to the wet ingredients. Wrap dough in plastic and chill until firm enough to roll.

Roll out dough on a GF flour covered surface. Cut out cookies and bake on greased sheets for 12 minutes, or until just golden at the edges. Cookies will be soft when they come out of the oven but will firm up a bit as they cool. For crispier cookies, bake a little longer, taking care not to burn them.

To decorate, use icing and small GF/CF candies, dried fruits and chocolate chips. Be sure to put on decorative items before the icing dries.

*Any GF flour mix will work, but my favorite for making cookies is 1 1/4 parts rice flour mixed with 3/4 part garfava flour (available from Authentic Foods). Be warned—garfava flour tastes terrible when raw so don't be tempted to sneak a little dough. The "beany" taste will bake out, however, and the extra protein in this flour makes it easier to roll out.

Mock Chopped Liver

This is a very strange recipe. It contains no meat and yet really tastes like traditional Jewish chopped liver. It is great on crackers and Sam loves it. It makes a nice appetizer for the grownups who are watching their cholesterol and would never dream of eating the real thing. If your kids eat it too, that's great.

I've seen versions of this recipe in lots of magazines—this is one I got from my mother, who has no idea where she got it. She has made it for years.

Ingredients

2 onions, chopped

5 hard-boiled eggs, whites only

1 cup chopped walnuts

1 8-ounce can of peas (drain but reserve liquid)

CF margarine or oil

Sauté the onions in oil or margarine until very brown.

Place onions, egg whites, walnuts and peas into a food processor or blender, using most of the liquid from the peas. If it seems dry, add the rest of the liquid. Season with salt and pepper and chill thoroughly.

Bean Flour Matzo

Passover matzo is always made from wheat, and I am often asked how to make it from other flours. I usually skip it, but this year Sam's teacher asked me to send in some matzo that Sam could eat. This recipe was originally a Bette Hagman pasta recipe, then was modified by Gina Levy and posted to the Yahoo group Gfcfrecipes (see appendix information on how to join).

Ingredients

1/3 cup tapioca starch

1/3 cup cornstarch plus additional for kneading

1/3 cup Garfava flour

1/2 teaspoon salt (optional)

2 teaspoons xanthan gum

1 tablespoon olive oil

2 eggs

In a medium bowl, combine the flours, salt and xanthan gum. Whisk together the eggs and the oil, pour into the dry ingredients and stir until a ball forms. Knead for a minute or two, adding more cornstarch if necessary.

Work in cornstarch until the dough will not accept any more and is firm. Place the ball on a cutting board dusted with cornstarch and roll as thin as possible. Cut into matzo board shapes and poke rows of holes with a fork.

Carefully lift onto an ungreased cookie sheet and bake at 400° for 8-10 minutes or until crispy.

Passover Rolls

These rolls are typically made with matzoh meal during the Jewish holiday of Passover. Since matzoh meal contains gluten, try making them with Paskez brand Pesach Crumbs®. These "crumbs" are made of potato starch and egg, and can be used for any recipe that calls for matzoh meal. They are available only in the passover season, so when spring comes, try finding them in a Kosher market. Or visit a website such as: **www.mykoshermarket.com.** *You can also try* **www.kosher.com.** *Note: both close several days before Passover, so shop early. If you cannot get them, try substituting ground Hol Grain crackers or Schär® brand GF cracker crumbs.*

Ingredients

1 1/2 cups water

1/4 cup safflower oil

1/2 teaspoon salt

2 1/4 cups Pesach crumbs

4 eggs

Preheat oven to 375°.

Bring water, oil and salt to a boil in a medium saucepan over medium-low heat. Remove from heat and add crumbs. Mix well.

Return pan to low heat and cook, stirring, for 1 minute; remove from heat and cool 5 minutes.

Place in mixer fitted with flat paddle; beat in one egg. When mixture is smooth, beat in second egg. Continue adding eggs one by one, beating after each addition.

Drop batter by heaping tablespoons (2 tablespoons to each roll), onto parchment-lined baking sheets, allowing about 1 1/2" between them.

Bake about 30-40 minutes, or until golden brown and firm.

Peanut Butter-Marshmallow Eggs

I don't celebrate Easter, but questions about Easter candy fill my email box every spring. There are many acceptable GF/CF candies out there, but I found a recipe for homemade candy eggs and realized that it could be modified to suit the GF/CF regime (definitely NOT a low sugar diet, however). If you are looking for a fun, homemade basket filler, this might be the recipe for you. After all, it's just once a year.

Ingredients

1 1/2 cups CF margarine, softened

6 cups confectioner's sugar*, sifted and divided

1 cup peanut butter (other nut butters should also work)

1 3/4 cups marshmallow cream**

2 teaspoons vanilla

1 3/4 lbs GF/CF chocolate, melted

Cream the margarine and 2 cups of the confectioners sugar in large bowl until light and fluffy. Add the nut butter, marshmallow cream and vanilla, blending well.

Gradually add remaining confectioner's sugar; mix to consistency that can be easily handled; form into egg shapes and dip in melted chocolate; let sit until firm.

*If sensitive to corn, be aware that most confectioner's sugar does contain cornstarch. You can buy corn-free powdered sugar during the Passover holidays. Be sure to stock up. You can also grind sugar yourself, if you have a good food processor.

**As of this writing Solo® marshmallow cream is GF, but be sure to read labels and call the company if in doubt.

Peppermint Stick Ice Cream

*My son got a taste of his dad's peppermint stick ice cream and went wild for it. I promised him I would make a **special** version for his 13th birthday and here it is.*

*This ice cream mixture is not cooked, so you may want to consider using dried eggs instead of fresh. Dried whole eggs are available from the King Arthur Flour Company. They also have lots of fabulous pans and other baking tools, so be sure to check them out at **www.bakerscatalogue.com**. Peppermint oil can be purchased from candy making stores, or use a GF peppermint extract.*

The candy makes this a very festive dessert and it would be great after a heavy holiday meal. Perfect for a Fourth of July picnic.

Ingredients:

1 large egg, or equivalent dried egg

4 cups DariFree liquid, very cold

3/4 cup granulated sugar

1 teaspoon peppermint oil or $1/4$ teaspoon peppermint extract

2-3 GF peppermint sticks, crushed (leave some small chunks)

Combine egg, sugar, peppermint oil and 1 cup DariFree in blender or food processor. Blend until smooth and then add the other 3 cups of DariFree. Blend well. Transfer mixture to ice-cream machine and freeze according to manufacturer's instructions. When ice cream is almost completely frozen, add candy.

Gefilte Fish

Homemade gefilte fish is a wonderful delicacy, usually served during Passover. It bears little resemblance to the stuff you can buy in jars, which also happens to contain matzo meal (and thus gluten).

If you have a food processor, and a market that stocks really fresh fish, it is not hard to make from scratch. It may not be something you'd do every day, but it really is good and well worth the trouble.

It is traditionally served with strong horseradish—the stronger the better—but that is most certainly optional. Instead of matzo meal, substitute finely ground Hol Grain rice crackers, or Glutano bread crumbs. If your family does not use grain during Passover, substitute Pesach crumbs.

Ingredients

2 lbs winter carp

2 lbs whitefish

2 quarts water

1 1/2 teaspoons pepper

3 carrots, sliced

2 lbs pike

5 onions

4 teaspoons salt

3 eggs

3 tablespoons GF bread or cracker crumbs

Have the fished filleted at the store but be sure you get the head, skin and bones.

Combine these "spare parts" with 4 of the onions (chopped), a quart of water, 2 teaspoons salt and 3 teaspoons pepper. Cover and cook over high heat while preparing your fish balls.

Grind or chop the fish and the remaining onion (a food processor works well if you don't have a grinder). Add the eggs, crumbs and remaining salt and pepper; process or grind all the ingredients until very fine.

Wet your hands and shape the fish mixture into balls. Drop the fish balls (gently) into the boiling fish stock. Add the carrots, then cover and cook over low heat for 1 1/2 hours.

Remove the cover for the last half-hour of cooking. Use a slotted spoon to remove the fish from the pot. Strain the broth and set aside to serve with the fish, if desired. Serve warm, room temperature or chilled. This is strictly a personal preference.

Chapter 7
Snacks & Goodies

*C*hildren generally have small appetites, so they rarely eat a great deal at any meal. Most nutritionists suggest frequent small meals rather than three squares a day, and that pattern certainly works best for small children. Preschoolers usually need a morning snack between breakfast and lunch, and at least one more snack before dinner.

School age children too will head to the refrigerator as soon as they get home. Fresh fruit and vegetables would make a good after-school snack, but of course many of our kids avoid these healthful alternatives.

Most children could also use a protein boost at this time of day, so even in the unlikely event that your kids will be happy with carrot sticks, be sure they have some nut butter to dip them in. Hard fruits like apples and pears also taste good smeared with a nut butter or tahini.

Sometimes you just need a little something more for that time between school and dinner. The recipes here will give you some additional choices. Most have a satisfying crunch, and nearly all have some protein. Experiment with ingredients your child likes, and don't forget to sneak in some calcium powder or ground flax seed whenever possible.

Nutty Crunch

Nuts make a terrific snack for small children who aren't yet worrying about their fat intake. They are a high-protein, high-energy food. Since children have small appetites, their protein intake is often not what it should be. A small serving of this crunchy treat will help.

Ingredients

5 cups Gorilla Munch Cereal

I cup roasted almonds

I cup raisins

I cup dried cherries

I small package vanilla pudding* (not instant)

1/2 cup honey

1/2 cup almond butter (or other nut butter)

Lightly butter a jellyroll pan. Mix first 4 ingredients in a large bowl.

Mix dry pudding mix and honey in a small saucepan. Heat to boiling over medium heat, stirring constantly. Reduce heat. Boil and stir I minute, then remove.

Stir in almond butter. Pour over cereal mixture; toss until evenly coated.

Spread in pan and refrigerate for 30 minutes.

Break into bite-size pieces. Store snack in covered container at room temperature or in refrigerator.

*Stock up on GF/CF pudding mixes around Passover.

Nut Bars

These delicious nut bars are packed with protein. If nuts are tolerated, they make a terrific snack. They lend themselves to flour substitution, so if you rotate grains, don't feel that sorghum is your only choice. Use whatever nuts your family likes and tolerates. A mixture of more than one kind of nut works very well.

Ingredients

1 1/2 cups sorghum flour

2 teaspoons xanthan gum

3/4 cup packed brown sugar

1/2 cup CF margarine or coconut butter, melted

1 12-ounce can (about 2 cups) salted nuts

1 cup GF/CF chocolate chips

1/2 cup corn syrup (use pure cane syrup if corn is not tolerated)

3 tablespoons ghee

In a medium bowl, combine flour, xanthan gum, brown sugar, and the 1/2 cup melted shortening (mixture will be crumbly). Press mixture into an ungreased 13 x 9 x 2-inch baking pan. Bake in a 350° oven for 12 minutes. Sprinkle nuts over baked crust.

In a small saucepan, heat chocolate chips, ghee and corn syrup over low heat, stirring to prevent burning. When melted, drizzle this mixture evenly over nuts.

Bake for 8 minutes more. Cut into bars while warm.

Crunch 'Ems Mix

It was such a boon to GF cereal lovers when Health Valley® introduced their "Crunch Em" line of products. Although the rice version contains a minute amount of cornstarch, they are well tolerated even by corn-allergic individuals and are worth a try. If corn intolerant, omit Corn Crunch Ems.

Ingredients

1 cup GF pretzels

6 tablespoons CF margarine

2 tablespoons GF Worcestershire sauce

1 1/2 teaspoons seasoned salt (see recipe page 223)

3/4 teaspoons garlic powder

1/2 teaspoon onion powder

3 cups Corn Crunch Ems® cereal

3 cups Rice Crunch Ems® cereal

1 cup mixed nuts (optional)

Preheat oven to 250°

Melt margarine in large roasting pan in oven. Stir in seasonings.

Gradually stir in remaining ingredients until evenly coated. Bake 1 hour, stirring every 15 minutes.

Spread on paper towels to cool. Store in airtight container.

Cereal Munch

Here's a sweet treat that would be appropriate around Halloween, when all the other kids are eating sweet, goopy treats. Use any nut that is tolerated, or omit nuts altogether if necessary. Be sure to read the label on the marshmallow bag carefully; some do not specify the type of starch used. It could be wheat. If corn-intolerant, stock up on Kosher corn-free marshmallows around Passover time. They will harden in time, even if well-wrapped but will still melt down for Crispie treats and recipes like this one.

Ingredients

3 cups puffed rice cereal

1 cup dried apricots; chopped

1 cup raisins

1 cup GF/CF chocolate chips

1 cup dry-roasted nuts

1/3 cup CF margarine

1 bag GF marshmallows

1/2 cup peanut butter (substitute if desired)

In a large bowl, combine cereal, apricots, raisins and peanuts. In microwave-safe 13 x 9 inch baking dish, melt margarine and marshmallows on high for 2 minutes. Stir. Add peanut butter. Cook on high 2 minutes longer. Stir until blended.

Add cereal mixture to dish. Toss until well coated.

Working quickly with greased hands, form into balls, using about 1/2 cup mixture per ball. If mixture begins to cool and harden, microwave on high 30 seconds or until softened.

Variation: Omit the peanut butter and margarine and just toss the ingredients together and you've got gorp.

Gorp

I'm not sure how trail mix came to be called gorp—some contend that it stands for Good Old Raisins and Peanuts. It's always a good idea to have some when you hit the trail, and sometimes I think it is the reason Sam likes to hike so much. Here's another recipe, but remember, anything you like is a good addition to gorp.

Ingredients

I cup roasted, salted nuts (your choice)

I cup raisins

I cup puffed rice

I cup sunflower seeds

I cup coconut (preferably sulfite free)

I cup dried apricots, chopped

I cup GF/CF chocolate "lentils"* or

I cup GF/CF chocolate chips

Mix all ingredients in a large bowl, then place in serving size plastic bags.

*M & Ms contain milk and are forbidden, but it is possible to find the same type of candy in a dairy free version. Check stores that have good supplies of Kosher foods. Bloomy's® is a brand that is widely available, but there are many others.

Raisin Snack Cake

*Ever since I read Louise Fitzhugh's **Harriet The Spy** when I was in fifth grade, I've loved the idea of cake and milk after school. This one is very simple and just sweet enough to be good. It's a great after school snack with a big glass of Darifree. It makes a good lunchbox addition too. I love to use dried fruits other than raisins when I bake, and usually have dried cherries, cranberries and blueberries on hand.*

Ingredients

1 cup raisins (or other dried fruit)

2 cups water

1/2 cup CF margarine

1 cup GF flour blend

3/4 cups sorghum flour

2 teaspoons xanthan gum

1/2 cup sugar

1/2 teaspoon salt

1 teaspoon baking soda

1 teaspoon cinnamon

1/2 teaspoon nutmeg (preferably freshly grated)

1 teaspoon vanilla

1/2 chopped nuts

Preheat oven to 350°.

Bring the water to a boil and add the raisins. Remove from heat and let the raisins "steep" for about 10 minutes, then cool. Combine all other ingredients with the water and fruit and mix well. Bake in 10 x10-inch pan for 30-35 minutes or until the cake tests done. If you use a loaf pan, increase the baking time to 50-55 minutes.

Date-Nut Bread

This quick bread hides carrots, and the nuts and eggs make it a nice protein-filled snack.

It's great toasted for breakfast, or serve plain for a snack. Add a teaspoon of calcium powder if you want to.

Ingredients

3/4 cup hot water

1/2 cup pitted dates, chopped

1/2 cup golden raisins

1 cup shredded carrot

1/2 cup coarsely chopped walnuts

3 tablespoons vegetable oil

2 large eggs

1 large egg white

2 cups GF flour blend

2 teaspoons xanthan gum

3/4 cup sugar

1 tablespoon baking powder

1 1/2 teaspoons ground cinnamon

1/2 teaspoon salt

Cooking spray

Preheat oven to 350°.

Combine water, dates, and raisins in a bowl; let stand 15 minutes.

Stir in carrot, walnuts, oil, eggs, and egg white. Combine flour, sugar, baking powder, cinnamon, and salt in a large bowl. Add carrot mixture to flour mixture, stirring just until moist. Spoon batter into an 8 x 4-inch loaf pan coated with cooking spray.

Bake for 1 hour or until a wooden pick inserted in center comes out clean. Cool 10 minutes in pan on a wire rack; remove from pan. Cool completely on wire rack.

Fruit Kebobs

Most children like fresh fruit, and what could be more fun than fruit on a stick? If you like, roll the finished kebobs in coconut just before serving. Messy, but good. This is a fun thing to bring to a picnic. If your kids are very little, beware of the pointy skewers.

Ingredients

Melon, cubed or scooped with a melon baller

Pineapple chunks

Seedless grapes

Apple, cubed

Pear, cubed

Strawberries, hulled

Lemon juice

Coconut

Clean all the fruit and cut into appropriate chunks. Thread thin bamboo skewers with fruit chunks to make kebobs. Sprinkle the finished kebobs with a little lemon juice if not serving immediately. Coat with coconut if desired.

Halvah

When I was in college I frequented a delicatessen called "Bubby and Zayde's" (Grandma and Grandpa's). They sold wonderful coffee and always had a huge brick of halvah, from which they chipped off small portions and sold them by weight. This recipe comes from Lundberg Family Farms, and uses their gluten-free rice syrup as its sweetener. When buying rice syrup, beware that most are not gluten-free, but Lundberg Farms does make one with "Gluten Free" on the label.

Ingredients

1/4 cup tahini

1/4 cup Lundberg Farms Gluten Free Rice Syrup

1 teaspoon grated orange or lemon rind (optional)

Pinch sea salt

1 cup finely ground GF crackers

1/4 cup toasted sesame seeds, slightly crushed, or toasted unsweetened
    coconut

Place tahini in a small skillet and roast over a low flame for 2 minutes, stirring constantly, until tahini changes color and develops a nutty aroma. With a spatula, scrape tahini into a small mixing bowl. Add rice syrup, citrus rind, and salt.

Mix well and stir in cracker crumbs. Roll by teaspoonfuls into balls and roll balls in sesame seeds or coconut. Store covered to prevent drying out, and serve as a snack. For a slightly sweeter treat, omit the cracker crumbs and use as a spread for crackers, rice cakes or slices of apple or pear.

Blueberry-Applesauce Fruit Leather

Fruit leather is a very chewy and delicious dried-fruit treat. The sugars, acids, fiber and nutrients found in fruit become concentrated when the water is removed. This makes dried fruits high in sugar, but the vitamins and mineral content is also high. Dried fruits provide a nutritious way to satisfy a sweet tooth.

Ingredients

Blueberries to make one cup of puree when blended

1 cup unsweetened applesauce

1 tablespoon honey

Combine all ingredients and spread evenly on plastic wrap. Dry fruit using a food dehydrator (follow manufacturer's instructions) or your oven.

Oven Dry: Set oven at 140°. Use an oven thermometer to test oven temperature. Too high a heat will disintegrate the plastic. Leave the oven door ajar so moisture can escape. It takes about 6 hours to dry fruit leather in the oven, but always test for dryness.

To make sure the fruit leather is completely dried, try to pull the leather from the plastic wrap. If it peels from the plastic and holds its shape, it is dry. Incompletely dried fruit will not keep well. When dry, roll fruit leather loosely in plastic wrap and place in an airtight container. They will keep for more than a year if refrigerated or frozen.

Frozen Banana Pops

I first experienced frozen bananas at the Dairy Queen when I was very young. I hear they still have them, though the area where I live doesn't have DQs. They are easy enough to make however, and fun to eat. If your child tolerates bananas they make a great summertime treat.

Ingredients

2 bananas

8 ounces GF chocolate chips

2 tablespoons Darifree (liquid)

1 tablespoon solid shortening

Peel and cut bananas in half and insert a skewer or stick.

In double boiler or microwave, melt chips with shortening and Darifree. Dip banana chunks into chocolate and cool on wax paper. When hardened, wrap well and freeze.

Puppy Chow

I won't try to kid anyone. There is nothing nutritious about this recipe, but boy-oh-boy is it ever good. Save it for very special treats, or perhaps those occasions when a bribe is needed. I have packaged this in nice jars and given it as teacher presents.

Ingredients

1/2 cup peanut or other nut butter

1/2 cup CF margarine

6 ounces GF/CF chocolate chips

10 cups Rice or Corn Crunch Ems cereal

2 cups powdered sugar

Melt peanut butter, butter or margarine, and chocolate chips in a saucepan over medium heat. Pour over cereal, being sure that all cereal is coated.

Put 2 cups powdered sugar in a large paper bag. Put cereal in bag and shake gently until all cereal is coated. Pour out on wax paper to cool.

Kiddie Kibbles

Everyone knows that the croutons are the best part of a salad. So why not just cut to the chase and snack on the croutons? I call these snacks kibbles because they remind me of my dog's crunchy food.

Ingredients

1 recipe GF Garlic Croutons (see recipe on page 218)

1/2 cup CF margarine, melted

2 teaspoons sesame seeds

1 teaspoon celery seeds

1 teaspoon salt

1 teaspoon sweet paprika

Preheat oven to 275°.

Pour croutons into large bowl. Combine remaining ingredients and toss with croutons. Place onto cookie sheet and toast for 20 minutes, stirring every 5 minutes. Allow to cool.

Ants on a Log

Your children have probably made these at school—nearly everyone does. They are fun to make and eat. Feel free to use a different nut butter, or if no nut is tolerated you can use tahini.

Ingredients

Celery stalks

Peanut butter

Raisins

Take a stalk of celery and fill center with peanut butter. Place raisins on top.

Variation: For a sweet treat, substitute maple butter for the nut butter.

"Caramel" Apple Slices

Caramel always contains milk—I have yet to find one that does not. I thought about making my own, but when I read caramel recipes I decided it was a little ambitious for most cooks (including me). This makes a good treat for those times when you just need a sweet. Pears can be used if apples are not tolerated. Nothing could be simpler and I can't really call this a recipe at all. Try this around Halloween, when the apples are tart and crisp, and everyone else is eating caramel apples.

Ingredients

Apples (or pears)

Maple Butter*

Slice fruit and spread with maple butter. Eat.

*Maple butter, despite its suspicious-sounding name, contains no dairy at all. In fact, it contains nothing but maple syrup, which has been cooked down to a thick, spreadable consistency. It is wonderful spread on toast or waffles and a real fall treat on fruit.

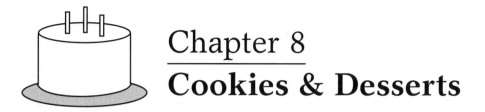

Chapter 8
Cookies & Desserts

As I said in **Special Diets for Special Kids,** we all eat too much sugar. Every year or so newspapers publish the amount of sugar the average American eats in a year, and the number is staggering. It is currently estimated that we each eat 150 pounds of sugar every year!

Sugar is not inherently evil. In my opinion, however, sweets have three major strikes against them.

First, they are empty calories. If a child eats very little to begin with or is extremely fussy, it is very hard to get the required nutrients into them on a daily basis. If they have used up some of their small capacity on empty calories, it is nearly impossible.

Second, many autistic spectrum children have a demonstrable overgrowth of yeast. Sugar feeds yeast, which after all are living organisms, so it must be strictly limited when trying to overcome this problem. Fortunately, in most cases a combination of diet, anti-fungal medication and probiotic supplements eventually defeats the yeast problem. For some the problem can be persistent however, and they really must avoid refined AND natural sugars for a time.

Finally, we all know our dentists hate sugar for the simple reason that it promotes tooth decay. The idea of trying to fill the teeth of many autistic spectrum children is enough to scare the sugar out of most homes!

All that said, however, sweets taste good and kids love them! I do believe that there is a place for sweets in the diet, albeit a small one. (Dieticians generally suggest that fewer than 10% of our daily calories come from sources of refined sugars.) For children who are *fighting a yeast problem, intake of sugars must be drastically lowered. In fact, without substantial modification, most of the recipes in this chapter will be inappropriate for those on an anti-yeast regimen. However, there are sweetening ingredients that don't promote the growth of yeast. These include:*

- *100% pure food grade vegetable glycerin*

- *Stevia*

- *Xylitol*

- *Splenda® (sucralose)*

Vegetable glycerin is a thick, sweet, viscous liquid that is derived from coconut and well tolerated by most people. It does not feed yeast and can be used to sweeten many foods. It is easiest to substitute with glycerin when the original recipes calls for a liquid sweetener such as honey, molasses or maple syrup. It is quite a bit sweeter than sugar, and you may have to experiment to get the amount right. If you do choose to use this liquid sweetener in a recipe that calls for regular sugar, you may need to decrease the liquid ingredients and add something to make up for the bulk of the missing sugar.

*Stevia is an herb **(stevia rebaudiana)** in the Chrysanthemum family. It grows wild as a small shrub in parts of Central and South America. The glycosides in its leaves, including up to 10% stevioside, account for its incredible sweetness. There are hundreds of species of stevia plants, but only the leaves of **S. rebaudiana** are used as a sweetener.*

Stevia comes in several forms. The white powdered extract or the liquid extract are likely to be most useful to you when preparing foods for your family. The green leaves are available in powdered form, but they tend to discolor food. All stevia can have a bitter aftertaste and if too much is used it will have a hint of licorice flavor. Many people who limit sugar have used stevia enthusiastically—I suggest you purchase a small amount at your local health food store and experiment. There are many recipes available at **www.stevia.com.** *You will learn how to modify your own family's favorites and some of the recipes in this chapter.*

Xylitol was discovered by a German chemist in 1891, and has been used as a sweetener in this country for nearly forty years. Refined to a white crystalline powder, xylitol is odorless, with a pleasant, sweet taste. It has gained increasing acceptance as an alternative sweetener due to its role in reducing the development of dental cavities, and is often used to sweeten chewing gum.

Produced commercially from plants such as birch and other hard wood trees, xylitol has the same sweetness and bulk as sugar with one-third fewer calories and no unpleasant aftertaste. This means that it can be used, cup for cup, as you would use sugar. It dissolves quickly and produces an odd, yet pleasant cooling sensation in the mouth.

Xylitol is sold in several forms and under many names. Miss Roben's sells a brand called "The Ultimate Sweetener" in both granular and powdered form. Xylitol is well tolerated by most people (though there are certainly people who are allergic to birch bark and they should not use it). It does not feed yeast and is appropriate for yeast-free diets.

Sucralose is an artificial sweetener developed at Johnson & Johnson and sold under the trade name of Splenda®. Like Nutrasweet®, many people believe it has received inadequate testing and others say avoid it and all artificial sweeteners completely. I think the jury is still out, but assume that, in very limited amounts, it would not be harmful.

When changing recipe ingredients, achieving just the right texture may take some experimentation. There are various ways to make up for the lost bulk, such as adding rice bran, apple fiber, ground flaxseeds, unsweetened coconut or calcium powder.

In general, if you are avoiding sugar in your family's diet, I would say that xylitol makes the best overall substitute. Because you can use it as a cup-for-cup substitute, adding extra bulk to a recipe is not necessary. On the down side, it is expensive, at approx-

imately $9.00/lb. However, if your child must be on a sugar-free diet, it is probably worth the expense to be able to provide an occasional cookie!

Experiment with substituting sugar alternatives in the recipes that follow and in your family's favorites. You may also want to use a combination of a little sugar and one of the substitutes. This will appreciably lessen the amount of sugar being consumed, while reducing any unusual flavor or aftertaste.

For really picky children, cookies and desserts present us with an opportunity for "sneaking in" nutrients that may otherwise be lacking in the diet. Growing children need between 800 and 1200 mg of calcium per day, for example, and for kids who don't eat or drink dairy it is sometimes hard to get in the required amount. Powdered calcium is easily added to any of the recipes in this booklet and I recommend you do so. A teaspoon of Kirkman Lab's powdered calcium contains 1332 mg. of this important mineral, and most recipes can take the addition of several teaspoons without a discernible change in texture. The powder is slightly sweet, however, so you may want to reduce your sweetener when using more than 1-2 teaspoons.

All children need the essential fatty acids (EFA), but few get them. Although flaxseed oil cannot be heated, ground flaxseed adds EFAs, as well as bulk and a delicious nutty flavor. If you are searching for even more ways to get added protein into the diet, most cookies can take an extra egg or two. Extra egg helps add moisture and holds together cookies. Raisins and other dried fruits add both sweetness and nutrients (e.g., iron in raisins, calcium in figs, etc.).

One last note about ingredients—I use a lot of peanut butter! It is a nutrient-dense food that most children love, and it adds moisture and fat to a recipe. I realize, however, that many kids cannot tolerate peanuts. Any nut butter will work in recipes that specify peanut butter. Remember that peanuts are legumes—a peanut intolerance does not mean that tree nuts are unacceptable (though for extremely allergic children they might not be appropriate). Don't forget to try the more unusual nut butters such as pistachio and macadamia. If you fear cross-contamination, it is simple to make your own nut butter if you have a blender with a strong motor or a good food processor. If your child cannot tolerate any nut, tahini paste often makes a good substitute. Made from sesame seeds, tahini adds a similar taste and texture and has the added benefit of being another source of calcium.

Sugar-Free Pineapple Velvet Cake

*Lynne Davis contributed Pineapple Velvet Cake to **Special Diets for Special Kids**, and it was a real hit with nearly everyone. Then a few months ago I read a posting to the GF/CF*

Recipes Online group, which claimed a "sugar free version of everyone's favorite." The posting was in response to another reader's plea for a birthday cake she could make for her GFCFYF child. Alicia Rumple was the creator of the recipe. Alicia's daughter had had nothing sweet for about six weeks when Alicia came up with this recipe. Her little girl ate three pieces at the first sitting!

Ingredients

1 1/2 cups GF Flour mix (Alicia uses sorghum, tapioca and potato starch)

1 teaspoon baking soda

3 teaspoons baking powder

1/2 teaspoon salt

4 eggs

1 cup oil

3/4 cup DariFree powder

1 teaspoon Stevia

2 teaspoons rice vinegar (or lemon juice)

3/4 cup unsweetened pineapple juice

1/4 cup club soda

Preheat oven to 350°.

Combine the first 5 ingredients and set aside. With an electric mixer, combine all other ingredients except the juice and club soda. Beat well so that the oil is fully emulsified. Turn mixer to low and add the flour mix and juice, alternating. When all is well mixed, add the club soda and beat just to combine. Pour batter into greased and floured cake pans and bake for 25 minutes.

Lisa Ackerman's Chocolate Cake

Lisa swears that no one will peg this one for gluten-free and I think she may be right. She modified it from one she got from the GFCFKids internet list. This recipe has another feature you'll appreciate—it can all be made in one bowl! Double the recipe to make two round cake layers or a sheet cake.

Ingredients

1 cup white rice flour

1/2 cup sorghum flour

1 cup sugar

1/2 cup cocoa powder

1/2 teaspoon salt

1 teaspoon baking soda

1 teaspoon xanthan gum

1/2 cup oil

1/2 cup milk substitute

1/2 cup hot water

2 teaspoons CF vanilla

Preheat oven to 350°.

Mix together dry ingredients and stir to combine. Then add liquid ingredients and stir until well mixed.

Pour batter into a greased and floured 8 x 8-inch cake pan. Bake for 30 minutes or until the cake tests done with a toothpick. (Bake 20-25 minutes for cupcakes.)

Chocolate Frosting

You don't have to frost the cake, but here's a nice dairy-free recipe should you decide to.

Ingredients

1/4 cup GF/CF margarine, softened

1/3 cup cocoa powder

1 teaspoon GF vanilla

2 cups confectioner's sugar

4 tablespoons water

Beat margarine until fluffy, and then lower mixer speed and beat in cocoa and vanilla. Gradually beat in sugar, alternating with water, until desired thickness is achieved.

Lemon Chiffon Pie

*When I was young, my mother used to make lemon chiffon pie from a Jello® package, and we all loved it. A few years ago I began to search for that stuff, and simply could not find it. I finally contacted the company, and was told that they stopped making it years ago. I was really excited to find a recipe for it that really tastes a lot like the one I remember. I included a recipe for lemon chiffon in **Special Diets for Special Kids,** but this one is different and is also corn-free.*

Ingredients

1 tablespoon unflavored gelatin

1/2 cup cold water

4 eggs, separated

1 cup sugar

1/2 cup lemon juice

1/2 teaspoon salt

1/2 teaspoon lemon oil*

Soften the gelatin in the cold water for about 5 minutes. Set aside.

Beat egg yolks with 1/2 cup sugar, lemon juice and salt. Cook in a double boiler until the mixture reaches the consistency of custard. Cool.

Beat egg whites until foamy, then gradually add 1/2 cup sugar and beat until stiff. Fold egg whites into cooled custard and pour into graham crust. Chill.

*Available from Williams-Sonoma or King Arthur Flour.

Variation: Use the coconut crust recipe on page 185.

Graham Cracker Crust

*Health Valley makes a wonderful ersatz graham cracker called Rice Bran Crackers. I included this recipe in the **Special Diets for Special Kids,** but repeat it here since it will be useful with so many fillings.*

Ingredients:

1 package Healthy Valley Rice Bran crackers

1/4 cup sugar

1/4 cup CF margarine, softened

1/2 teaspoon cinnamon (optional)

Use a blender or processor to grind crackers into fine crumbs.

Combine all ingredients in a large mixing bowl. Mix until well blended.

Place crumbs into a 9-inch pie pan and press into the bottom and up the sides of the pan.

Bake crust at 350° for 6-8 minutes, until slightly toasted.

Cool slightly before spooning in cooked pie filling.

Variation: Pecan or almond meal enhance a graham crust.

Coconut Pie Crust

I adore coconut and use it whenever I can. This pie is delicious and uses no flour at all.

Be sure to use toasted coconut for the crust (see directions on page 215 for toasting coconut). This makes an excellent crust for any "cream" type pie.

Ingredients

2 1/2 cups shredded, unsweetened coconut, toasted

2 ounces GF/CF chocolate chips

4 tablespoons CF margarine, melted

In a small saucepan, melt the chocolate chips with the margarine. Combine toasted coconut with the chocolate. Refrigerate the mixture for 15 minutes, stirring every 5 minutes. When cool enough to handle, pat this mixture into a 9-inch glass pie pan and return to the refrigerator for at least 30 minutes.

Fill with the pudding or custard type pie filling and chill.

Taterdoodles

This is a very strange recipe that first appeared in my booklet "Gluten-Free Cookie Magic" (available through ANDI) It makes a surprisingly good cookie.

Ingredients

1/2 cup GF/CF margarine

1 1/2 cups GF flour mix

1 egg

1 1/2 teaspoons vanilla

1 1/4 cups potato flakes

1 cup sugar (or xylitol)

1 1/2 teaspoons baking powder

1 teaspoon xanthan gum

1 teaspoon cinnamon (optional)

Preheat oven to 350°.

Cream together margarine, sugar, egg and vanilla. Add flour, baking powder and xanthan gum. Mix well.

Fold in potato flakes.

Drop by teaspoon on lightly greased cookie sheet and bake for 12 minutes, or until lightly browned.

Choco-Nutty Crispy Bars

When I was growing up, my best friend's mom made the best Rice Krispie© treats in the whole world. Even Mrs. Shafer never thought of adding peanut butter, or of using the chocolate version of the cereal! It took Kellogg to think of that. Here is a GF/CF version of these popular treats. Note: Kellogg's version has a chocolate topping—I figure that is "gilding the lily" and I have left it off.

Ingredients

1 tablespoon CF margarine

3 tablespoons peanut or other nut butter

1/8 teaspoon salt

5 cups marshmallows*

1/2 teaspoon vanilla

6 cups New Morning Cocoa Crisp cereal

12-ounce bag dairy free chocolate chips**

Non-stick cooking spray

Combine margarine, nut butter and salt in a large saucepan over low heat. When nut butter and margarine have melted, add marshmallows and vanilla and stir until marshmallows have melted. Remove from heat.

Add cereal and stir until well coated with the marshmallow mixture.

Spray a 9 x 13-inch baking dish with a light coating of non-stick cooking spray.

Pour the cereal mixture into the dish and, using wax paper or lightly greased hands, press down until it's flat in the dish. Cool. Slice into approximately 16 bars.

*If the ingredients say "modified food starch" do not use unless you can verify that it is a gluten free source. If corn sensitive, note that Kosher, corn free marshmallows are available for the Jewish holiday of Passover (generally in March or April). Even when unopened, marshmallows do harden, but they should still melt, so stock up.

**Kellogg's uses milk chocolate chips, so CF chips will make a slightly different bar. They are still really good, however. Again, Passover is an excellent time to find dairy free and corn free chips.

Ice Cream Sandwiches

Every kid loves ice cream sandwiches, and being gluten free doesn't mean you can't have them. This recipe was adapted from two different chocolate cookie recipes—it stays soft and chewy so that the "ice cream" doesn't squish out when you eat it. I even had a rectangular cookie cutter made for me, but you can either make round sandwiches, or use a knife to cut them out. Using a fork to make a pattern of holes will keep the cookies from puffing too much, and it adds authenticity!

Ingredients

1 stick margarine (not tub)

1 cup brown sugar

2 eggs

1 teaspoon vanilla

1/2 cup cocoa powder

1 1/2 cup GF flour mix

1/2 cup Garfava flour

2 teaspoons xanthan gum

1 teaspoon baking powder

1/4 teaspoon salt

Sorbet, soy ice cream, or use one of the recipes that follow.

Cream the margarine and brown sugar, and then beat in the eggs, one at a time. Add vanilla.

Sift the cocoa, flour, xanthan gum and salt. Gradually add dry ingredients to the margarine-sugar mixture and beat until well combined. Gather the dough into a ball and wrap in plastic wrap. Chill the dough until it can be rolled out.

Preheat the oven to 375°.

Roll out the dough on a GF flour covered surface. Use a ruler and knife to cut out rectangular pieces (or use a round cookie cutter). Transfer the cookies to an ungreased cookie sheet. Use a fork to make the holes.

Bake for 8-10 minutes. The cookies will look "set." Cool before filling.

There are two approaches to ice cream sandwich assembly, so you can do whatever works best for you.

1. Soften the sorbet or soy ice cream. Use a spoon to place filling on the underside of one cookie, keeping it to the center. Place a second cookie on top and press just hard enough to spread the filling to the edges. Wrap in plastic and freeze until the whole sandwich is firm enough to hold.

OR

2. Freeze the sorbet or soy ice cream until very hard. Use the same cutter you used for making the cookies to cut out rounds or rectangles of ice cream. Place on a plastic lined cookie sheet and return to the freezer until firm. Place frozen ice cream in between two cookies, wrap in plastic and freeze.

Really Creamy, Really Rich Chocolate Ice Cream

Diane Hartman created this recipe and the two that follow. Jay Berger of Miss Roben's then modified these recipes. The directions specify how to make the ice cream without an ice cream machine, but if you have one, follow the manufacturer's directions. Visit Miss Roben's website for lots of other wonderful recipes created by Diane and others (see Appendix IV for more information.)

Ingredients

1 cup plus 2 tablespoons Chocolate DariFree powder

3/4 cup powdered confectioner's sugar

1 1/2 cups very hot water

2 tablespoons Spectrum Palm Shortening

1/2 tablespoon guar gum

Blend all ingredients well in a blender before pouring into a plastic, tightly lidded container. Place in freezer until frozen. Alternatively, prepare in any ice cream maker following manufacturer's instructions.

Super Strawberry Ice Cream

This is the result of another collaboration between Diane Hartman and Jay Berger, and it really is a treat. The last time I made it, unexpected company came while it was still mixing in my ice cream maker. I quickly added Rich's Rich Whip ® to stretch it for a few extra servings. It was as delicious as any regular ice cream I have had. If your child tolerates corn, and you can find Rich's, be sure to add ¹/2 cup. You can also use Kosher Parve whipping "cream," but again, it contains corn products.   I made this in my Krups Ice Cream maker.

Ingredients

1 ¹/2 cups fresh strawberries

1 cup DariFree powder

1 cup powdered confectioner's sugar

1 cup very hot water

2 tablespoons Spectrum Palm Shortening

¹/4 teaspoon vanilla extract

¹/2 tablespoon guar gum

[Up to 1 cup Rich's Rich Whip® or Hadar Parve Cream®]

Blend all ingredients well in a blender before pouring into a plastic, tightly lidded container.   Place in freezer until frozen. Alternatively, prepare in any ice cream maker following manufacturer's instructions.

Top Banana Ice Cream

The last in the Hartman-Berger trilogy, and the one that Jay's toddler likes best.

Ingredients

4 medium sized, ripe bananas

1 cup DariFree powder

1 cup powdered confectioner's sugar

1 cup very hot water

2 tablespoons Spectrum Palm Shortening

1/4 teaspoon vanilla extract

1/2 tablespoon guar gum

Blend all ingredients well in a blender before pouring into a tightly-lidded plastic container. Place in freezer until frozen. Alternatively, prepare in any ice cream maker following manufacturer's instructions.

Peaches & Cream Ice Cream

Diane created this one without modifications. It's a good way to bring a little summer back into the kitchen, even after the fresh peaches are just a distant memory.

1 can peaches with juice (use unsweetened if corn allergic)

2/3 cup DariFree powder or equivalent

1/2 cup cold water

1/4 cup oil

1 teaspoon safe vanilla extract (or use vanilla flavored sugar, if preferred)

1/2 cup granulated sugar, plus 1 cup hot water

In a saucepan, combine sugar and water. Bring to a boil and cook until dissolved. Cool. Transfer all ingredients into blender container, and process on high speed for 1 minute. Transfer mixture into the canister of ice cream maker and process according to manufacturer's instructions. If firm ice cream is desired, place ice cream into sealed freezer safe container and freeze for an additional 1-2 hours.

Orange Sorbet

Sorbets are easy to find at the grocery store, but if your family avoids corn you will have to make your own. Fortunately, they are simple to prepare if you have an ice cream maker.

Ingredients

1 cup simple syrup (equal parts sugar and water, boiled until sugar is dissolved)

1 cup orange juice

1/4 cup water

1 teaspoon lemon juice

In a small saucepan, heat the simple syrup to a simmer. Allow the syrup to cool to room temperature, then mix in the orange juice, water and the lemon juice. Freeze according to manufacturer's instructions.

For great information that will help you make terrific dairy free frozen desserts, see Appendix IV

Panda Puff Chocolate Crisps

First, Envirokiz® came up with Gorilla Munch cereal, and now they've given us Panda Puffs. This recipe makes delicious cookies. I first made them with Gorilla Munch, but since Panda Puffs are already peanut butter flavored, it was a natural. Of course, you can use Gorilla Munch and a different nut butter if necessary.

Ingredients

1/2 cup peanut butter

1/3 cup granulated sugar

1/3 cup packed brown sugar

1/3 cup CF margarine, softened

1/2 teaspoon baking soda

1/2 teaspoon baking powder

1 egg

4 cups Envirokiz® Panda Puffs cereal

1 cup GF semisweet chocolate chips

Heat oven to 325°.

Stir peanut butter, sugars, margarine, baking soda, baking powder and egg in large bowl until well mixed. Stir in cereal and chocolate chips. Shape dough by rounded tablespoonfuls into balls; place about 2 inches apart on ungreased cookie sheet (don't crowd them as these cookies tend to spread).

Bake 10 to 12 minutes or until golden brown. Cool 5 minutes; remove from cookie sheet. Cool completely. Store loosely covered.

Powdered Coolios [Sugar-free]

This cookie has a nice texture and is easy to make. Because it is made with powdered xylitol, you get a funny little cooling in your mouth when you eat them. Delicious AND fun.

Ingredients

I cup CF margarine, softened

I cup powdered xylitol

2 cups GF flour blend

1/2 teaspoon baking soda

I egg

I teaspoon GF vanilla

2 teaspoons xanthan gum

Preheat oven to 350°.

Cream margarine until fluffy. Beat in sugar then egg, and vanilla. Add flour, baking soda, xanthan gum and mix.

Shape dough into one-inch balls and arrange 2" apart on a lightly greased cookie sheet. Flatten with the tines of a (wet) fork. Bake 10-12 minutes until light brown.

Quick Brown Rice Fritters

*The people at Lundberg Family Farms produce dozens of excellent rice varieties and products. Their webpage (**www.lundberg.com**) has lots of interesting ideas for cooking rice. This recipe is very different and quite tasty. You could leave out the sweetening and substitute spices and serve it as a side dish instead of a dessert.*

Ingredients

2 cups cooked Lundberg Short Grain Brown Rice

1/2 cup sugar

3 eggs, beaten

1/2 teaspoon salt

1/4 teaspoon vanilla

6 tablespoons GF flour

1/2 teaspoon nutmeg

3 teaspoons baking powder

Combine rice, eggs, vanilla, nutmeg and mix well. Sift dry ingredients together and stir into rice mixture. Drop by spoonfuls into hot deep fat (360°) and fry until brown. Drain on absorbent paper, sprinkle with powdered sugar and serve hot. Makes 18 to 20 fritters.

Pudding Biscuits

In England, a biscuit is a cookie. These cookies are suitable for high tea, or at least an after-school snack!

Ingredients

3/4 cup GF/CF margarine, softened

1 cup sugar

1 egg

1 teaspoon baking powder

1 3-ounce package GF/CF instant pudding* (any flavor)

3 tablespoons tapioca starch

1 3/4 cup flour

2 teaspoons xanthan gum

Preheat oven to 350°.

Cream margarine and sugar; add egg and mix.   Mix in instant pudding and other dry ingredients. Drop by rounded teaspoonfuls onto ungreased cookie sheet. Flatten each cookie with a cookie stamp or the bottom of a drinking glass dipped in sugar.

Bake for 12 - 15 minutes or until the edges start to brown. Remove to wire rack to cool.

*Stock up on GF/CF corn-free pudding mixes during Passover.

Vanilla Cookies

This is a very simple cookie, not too sweet. They are reminiscent of the Vanilla Wafers you ate as a child. Be sure to flatten the cookies before baking.

Ingredients

1/2 cup powdered sugar

1/3 cup granulated sugar

1/3 cup shortening (Spectrum Palm shortening)

1 egg

1/2 teaspoon salt

2 teaspoons vanilla

1 1/2 cups GF flour

1 teaspoon xanthan gum

1 1/2 teaspoon baking powder

1 tablespoon water (if necessary)

Preheat oven to 325°.

Cream together the sugars, shortening, egg, vanilla and salt. Add flour, xanthan gum and baking powder. Beat until the dough comes together—if necessary add the water—and continue to mix until you can gather the dough into a ball. The dough should have the consistency of very fresh Play Doh.®

Roll the dough into very small balls and flatten to a wafer with the bottom of a sugar-dipped glass or cookie stamp. Bake for 15-18 minutes, until cookies are golden brown.

Crumb Bars

If cutting back on sugar, use powdered xylitol instead of confectioner's sugar and sweet, mashed peaches in place of jam. Grinding the nuts means that children who can tolerate nuts but don't like them, will get the nutritional benefit without knowing they are eating nuts.

Ingredients

1/2 cup GF flour blend

1/2 cups sorghum flour

1 cup GF/CF margarine

2 teaspoons xanthan gum

1 teaspoon additional GF flour

1/2 cup nuts, finely ground*

1/2 cup confectioner's sugar

3/4 cup jam or preserves

1 teaspoon cinnamon

1/2 cup toasted coconut

Preheat oven to 375°.

Combine flour and ground nuts and set aside.

In a large bowl, beat margarine until soft and then add powdered sugar. Beat until fluffy.

Combine the two mixtures and beat until it forms a dough.

Press 2/3 of the dough on to the bottom of an ungreased 8-inch square pan. Spread jam or fruit on top of the dough.

Combine 1-2 tablespoons of GF flour, coconut and the cinnamon to the remaining 1/3 of the dough. Mix with your hands or a fork to form a crumbly streusel. Sprinkle this mixture over the fruit and bake for 25-30 minutes. Cut into bars when still warm.

*Sesame seeds can be substituted for nuts.

Lemon Bars

I love lemon bars and just about every cookbook has a recipe for them. This one is particularly easy, because the filling is made in a blender rather than cooked (like a custard).

Ingredients

1/2 cup CF margarine, softened

1 1/3 cup GF flour blend

1 1/2 teaspoon xanthan gum

2 eggs

3/4 cup sugar

2 tablespoons tapioca starch

1/4 teaspoon GF baking powder

3 1/2 tablespoons lemon juice

1/4 cup confectioner's sugar

Preheat oven to 350°.

Mix together margarine, flour, sugar and xanthan gum. Use a pastry blender to work in the margarine until it is evenly distributed. The mixture will be crumbly. Press dough into a greased, 8-inch square pan and bake for 20 minutes. It will not brown.

Mix the remaining ingredients in a blender. Pour over the pre-baked crust and bake for another 20 minutes.

Cool and sprinkle with powdered sugar. Cut into bars when completely cool.

DAN! Cookies

*When the DAN! conferences were held in Cherry Hill, NJ, I used to make GF cookies to give out at the ANDI table. In 1999, these cookies caused a sensation and I had to promise to publish the (ridiculously simple) recipe in **The ANDI News.** I did, and I offer it to you here. If peanuts are ok for your child, these are definitely going to be a big hit.*

Ingredients

1/4 cup peanut butter (preferably chunky style)

2 eggs

1 cup GF chocolate chips (optional)

3/4 cup Jif Chocolate Silk Smooth Sensations

1 cup sugar

Preheat oven to 350°.

Combine all ingredients. Drop by teaspoon on greased or parchment-lined sheets. Bake for approximately 10 minutes or until lightly browned. Cool on racks and watch these disappear! If peanuts aren't tolerated, use 1 cup of another nut butter and add GF chocolate syrup to taste.

Rocky Road Bars

For the chocolate lovers in your family. Be sure to check the label of your marshmallows carefully; not all are gluten free. If your child is corn-intolerant, stock up on corn-free ones whenever you see them (e.g. around Passover.)

Ingredients

1/4 cup GF flour blend

1 teaspoon xanthan gum

1 cup ground nuts (walnuts or hazelnuts are best)

1/4 teaspoon baking powder

1/3 teaspoon salt

3 tablespoons CF margarine or coconut butter

1/3 cup brown sugar, packed

1 teaspoon GF vanilla extract

1 cup GF miniature marshmallows

1 cup GF chocolate chips

1 egg

Preheat oven to 350°.

Sift together dry ingredients (except nuts) and set aside.

In a medium bowl, beat together sugar, egg, margarine and vanilla. Stir in dry ingredients, and then add half of the ground nuts. Spoon batter onto greased 9-inch jellyroll pan.

Bake for 15 minutes and remove from oven. Sprinkle remaining nuts, chocolate chips and marshmallows evenly over the pan, then return to the oven for 5 minutes or until the chocolate is soft. Swirl the chocolate with a knife, and then cool until it sets. Cut into squares.

Apple Crisp

This crisp topping could be used for other fruits too, and the sugar can be cut back if desired.

Ingredients

1/2 cup GF flour blend

1/2 cup brown sugar

1 teaspoon xanthan gum

1 teaspoon cinnamon

1/2 cup CF margarine, cold

2 cups New Morning Crispy Rice Cereal (GF at time of writing)

8 cups apples, peeled and sliced

Preheat oven to 375°.

Combine flour, xanthan gum, sugar and cinnamon in a medium bowl. Cut in margarine with a pastry blender until the mixture is crumbly and the margarine evenly distributed.

Place apple slices in a 13 x 9-inch baking pan. Sprinkle topping over fruit and bake for 35-40 minutes or until apples are tender.

Demon Dogs

OK, so you can't eat Drake's Devil Dogs® on this diet, but there's no reason you can't make something similar that your kids will love. And there is no reason that they have to take a lot of work or time either. Use a good GF/CF chocolate cake mix like those sold by Miss Roben's, the Gluten Free Pantry or Authentic Foods. Because the cake will not be full of artificial colorings, your dogs will look different but the taste will be pretty darn close. If you can find a ladyfinger pan (check kitchen supply stores) it will make this recipe much easier. For best results, wrap each dog individually and freeze. A frozen, wrapped "dog" tossed into a lunchbox will be perfect by 11:15 a.m. (when most little kids eat lunch!).

Ingredients

1 package GF/CF chocolate cake mix

2 cups GF/CF marshmallow cream (7-ounce jar)

1 cup Spectrum® Shortening

1/2 cup powdered sugar

1/2 teaspoon vanilla

1/3 teaspoon salt dissolved in 2 teaspoon hot water

Preheat oven to 350°.

Prepare cake mix according to package directions.

For an authentic appearance, spoon batter onto a greased (or parchment lined) cookie sheet in 4-inch long strips. The strip should be about an inch wide.

Bake for about 5 minutes or until the cakes are done. Cool slightly then remove carefully from the pan.

To make the filling, combine the rest of the ingredients and beat with an electric mixer until light and fluffy.

To assemble, spread about a tablespoon of filling on half the cakes and top with a second one.

Variation: Use the batter to make cupcakes. When cupcakes are cooled, use a straw to make a small hole in the bottom of each. The hole should extend no more than $1/3$ through the cupcake. Using a pastry bag, inject cake openings with filling. To make it look like a Hostess Cupcake[®], frost cakes with chocolate frosting and pipe a white frosting squiggle on top!

Chocolate Wafers

This recipe is a great one if you want to recreate two all-time favorite cookies. The wafer can be filled and sandwiched with créme filling to make an Oreo® type cookie that your family will love. Alternatively, you can dip it and make a Thin Mint® cookie that will rival anything the neighborhood girls are hawking.

Ingredients

1 GF/CF chocolate cake mix

3 tablespoons solid shortening, melted

1/2 cup GF flour blend

1 egg

1/4 cup water

Combine ingredients in a large bowl, adding the water a little at a time until the dough forms. Gather dough into a ball, wrap tightly and refrigerate for at least 2 hours.

Preheat oven to 350°.

On a GF flour covered surface, roll out dough, a portion at a time, to no thicker than 1/16 inch. You want very thin cookies! Cut into very small cookies, 1 1/2-inch diameter (if you don't have a cutter that small, use the lid from a spice jar).

Bake cookies on a lightly greased cookie sheet for approximately 10 minutes.

To Make Mock Oreos®

Make the Demon Dog filling but omit the salt and reduce the shortening to $^1/_2$ cup.

When cookie wafers are cool, roll a small portion (about $^1/_4$ teaspoon) of the filling into a ball just over $^1/_4$-inch in diameter. Place it on the bottom of one cookie, cover with a second cookie and press them together to spread the filling to the edges of the sandwich.

To Make Thin Mints®

Melt a 12 ounce bag of GF/CF chocolate chips with 1 tablespoon shortening. When completely melted, add a few drops of peppermint oil (not extract) and stir well. Peppermint oil can be found in cake and candy making supply stores; it is very strong so do not use more than a couple of drops!

Using a fork (or special dipping tool available in candy making supply stores) dip each cookie into the chocolate. Let the excess drip off and place cookies on wax paper. When the chocolate hardens enough to touch the cookies, place them on wax paper covered cookie sheets and chill until completely firm. Wrap well and store in the refrigerator or freezer.

Coconut Macaroons

This macaroon recipe is easy and good. You don't need to, but these will look much nicer and be more uniform in size and shape if you pipe them from a pastry bag. Alternatively, place the mixture in a sealed plastic bag, and cut off one corner of the bag. Squeeze the mixture through the corner. Parchment paper is a must for macaroons, or you will not get them off the pan in one piece!

Ingredients

2 egg whites

1/2 cup sugar

3 tablespoons GF flour blend

1/3 teaspoon salt

1/4 teaspoon vanilla

1 1/3 cup coconut

Preheat oven to 350°.

Beat egg whites until foamy, then continue beating while you add the sugar very gradually. Beat until stiff and carefully fold in remaining ingredients. Pipe on to a parchment lined cookie sheet and bake for 12-15 minutes.

Variation: If desired, you can dip the bottoms of cooled macaroons in melted chocolate. Place upside down until chocolate hardens.

Peanutty Candy Bars

For this recipe, you really have to be able to eat corn and peanuts because substitutes just won't cut it. This will definitely remind you of Baby Ruth® bars, and should be saved for occasions like Halloween, when candy-eating is just about mandatory!

Ingredients

1 cup peanut butter

1 cup corn syrup

1/2 cup brown sugar, packed

1/2 cup sugar

6 cups GF cornflakes

1 cup GF chocolate chips

1/3 cup peanuts (roasted and salted)

Combine sugars, syrup and peanut butter in a saucepan and heat until smooth, taking care not to burn mixture. Add chocolate and stir until mostly melted. Stir in cereal and peanuts and mix well. Gently press mixture into a greased 9 x 13-inch pan. Cut into bars when cool.

Rolled Coconut Cookies

Here's another recipe that uses toasted coconut. The dough rolls out easily and can be cut into any shape you like.

Ingredients

1 cup lightly toasted, flaked coconut, cooled

1 cup sugar

2 1/4 cups GF flour

2 teaspoons xanthan gum

3/4 cup GF/CF margarine, cut into chunks

2 large eggs

1/2 teaspoon vanilla extract

2 tablespoons milk substitute

In a food processor, combine coconut and sugar. Process until coconut is coarsely ground. Pour the coconut/sugar mixture into a medium-size mixing bowl.

Combine flour, xanthan gum and margarine in the processor; process until the mixture is well blended and reduced to fine crumbs, about 30 seconds. Add the flour mixture to the coconut mixture. Stir to combine.

Add the eggs and vanilla. Knead to combine. If the mixture seems dry and does not form a dough, add up to 2 tablespoons milk substitute over ingredients until a dough forms. Put dough into a larger plastic container and refrigerate for 30 minutes.

Preheat oven to 375°.

Lightly grease two large baking sheets or line them with parchment paper. Generously flour the work surface and rolling pin. Remove half the dough, and refrigerate the remaining half.

Roll the dough to $1/4$-inch thickness and cut out with cookie cutters. Transfer to prepared baking sheets, keeping cookies at least 1-inch apart.

Form scraps into a ball and chill. Roll and cut remaining dough scraps. Bake one sheet at a time, 8 to 10 minutes. Cool on baking sheet for 5 minutes.

Chocolate Fudge

My friend Barbara Crooker sent me this recipe. It is, like all fudge, intensely sweet, so you should save it for very occasional treats. It is a favorite with her teenage son, Dave.

Ingredients

2 pounds confectioner's sugar

1 cup cocoa

$1/2$ cup milk substitute

1 cup CF margarine or $3/4$ cup coconut butter

2 tablespoons vanilla

1 $1/2$ cup walnuts, chopped

Combine sugar and cocoa in a large glass bowl. Add milk substitute and margarine and microwave on high for 3 minutes.

Add shortening and microwave for 3 minutes more.

Stir in vanilla then beat mixture until very smooth. Stir in walnuts and pour the mixture into a greased 13 x 9-inch pan. Chill completely then cut into (very small) squares.

Pizelles

These Italian cookies are always made in an appliance called a Pizelle Iron. While it is by no means a necessity, if you should happen to run across one at a garage sale pick it up! Pizelles make wonderful little cookies that are pliable when first removed from the iron, then harden as they cool. While they're hot they can be shaped into cones for ice cream, left flat to eat as is, or filled with ice cream, or molded (over the back of a custard cup) into an edible "dish." Experiment with different flavorings.

Ingredients

3 eggs

1 3/4 cup GF flour

3/4 cups sugar

1 tablespoon vanilla (or other flavoring)

1/2 cup margarine, melted (don't substitute with oil)

2 teaspoon baking powder

Beat eggs, adding margarine and vanilla. Add sugar gradually and then beat until smooth.

Sift GF flour and baking powder. Mix with egg mixture until smooth.

Bake pizelles for about 90 seconds on a preheated pizelle iron.

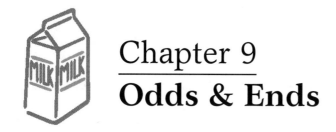

Chapter 9
Odds & Ends

*T*he recipes in this chapter do not fall easily into any category, or they are used in recipes throughout the book. Although they are stuck at the end, many are recipes you will want to try.

Evaporated Milk Substitute

Recipes often call for evaporated milk. Evaporated milk starts out as plain milk; a vacuum process evaporates about half the volume of water and concentrates the nutritive part of the milk. The evaporated milk is then poured into cans and heat-sterilized to prevent spoilage. The ultra-high temperatures of sterilization cause the milk sugars to caramelize and gives evaporated milk its characteristic cooked taste and color. In the end, evaporated milk has the consistency of light cream and a pale amber color.

Ingredients

1 cup DariFree powder

3/4 cup water

Combine DariFree and water in a blender. This condensed milk will not have the characteristic color of condensed milk, but will work well in recipes that call for it.

Sweetened Condensed Milk

Sweetened condensed milk is the same as evaporated milk, except that it has a LOT of sugar added to it! That is why it is used primarily in dessert recipes.

Ingredients

1 cup DariFree (or other milk substitute) powder

1 cup sugar

1 cup boiling water

1 tablespoon melted GF/CF margarine (optional)

1/2 teaspoon GF vanilla

Combine well in a blender. It will not be as thick as the store bought, canned evaporated milk, but should work in most recipes.

Ricotta Cheese Substitute

If your child can tolerate soy, this will make a good addition to casseroles and other dishes that call for ricotta or cottage cheese.

Ingredients

1 pound firm tofu, halved

1 cup safflower or other oil

1/2 teaspoon salt

Pinch of sugar (if tolerated)

Combine half the tofu with other ingredients and blend or process until smooth. Add the second half of the tofu and mash with a fork, leaving small curds.

Toasted Coconut

Many recipes call for toasted coconut. Even recipes that call for plain coconut can generally be improved by using toasted instead. Toasting brings out a wonderful aroma, flavor and a little bit of crunch.

Ingredients

Unsweetened coconut shreds

Preheat oven to 350°.

Spread coconut in shallow pan. Bake 10-20 minutes, stirring occasionally to make sure it toasts evenly. The goal is an even, dark golden. A few minutes too long and it will burn. Cool completely before storing in an airtight container at room temperature, and try to use within a few days.

Dumplings

Use Quickie Baking Mix to make these super simple dumplings.

Ingredients

2 cups Quickie Baking Mix

2 cups milk substitute

Combine ingredients and stir until a soft dough forms. Drop by spoonfuls onto boiling stew. Reduce heat and cook uncovered for 10 minutes. Cover and cook an additional 10 minutes.

Quickie Baking Mix

A General Mills® sales executive first got the idea for a quick baking mix back in 1930, and Bisquick® was the result. A staple of American kitchens for decades, it is of course off limits to those who cannot eat gluten. That's why I was so excited to try out Sue Crosby's alternative. (Sue is allergic to milk, and she has two kids with celiac disease.) This recipe is great! I have used it to create knock-offs of many of the wonderful recipes developed for the original, gluten-filled mixture. These include recipes for biscuits, pancakes, "Danish" pastry and Impossibly Easy® pies. I keep a large container of this mixture in my refrigerator at all times, and once you have tried it, I think you will too. Sue's version uses cornstarch, but if you are avoiding corn you can substitute tapioca starch or arrowroot starch.

Ingredients

10 cups GF flour*

3/8 cup baking powder

1 teaspoon cream of tartar

1 1/4 cups powdered milk substitute (DariFree or Better Than Milk soy powder)

1 1/2 tablespoons salt

1/4 cup sugar

1 pound shortening (Crisco or Spectrum solid shortening)

3 tablespoons xanthan gum

Mix all together and store in an airtight container. You will need to use a pastry blender or two knives to break up all the larger lumps. This will last for several months if kept in a tightly sealed, refrigerated container. The recipe can be halved, but why would you? It is so handy to have around!

*The flour combination that I have had great success with is:

   3 ^{1}/3 cups cornstarch

   3 ^{1}/3 cups tapioca flour (starch)

   2 cups garbanzo flour or bean flour mixture

   1 ^{1}/3 cups sorghum flour

Biscuits

And another "quickie" recipe.

Ingredients

2 ^{1}/4 cups Quickie Baking Mix

^{2}/3 cup milk substitute

Preheat oven to 450°.

Combine ingredients and stir until a dough forms. Place dough on a GF flour covered counter and knead dough until it is smooth. Roll dough out to a thickness of ^{1}/2 inch. Cut with a biscuit cutter or the bottom of a glass (approx. 2 ^{1}/2 inches in diameter).

Bake on ungreased cookie sheet about 10 minutes or until light brown.

Gluten Free Garlic Croutons

I know that most little kids don't eat salad, but croutons are also great tossed on soup. They make a good snack too. You can use leftover bread to make croutons of course, but I prefer using GF English Muffins because they are thick enough to cut into cubes. My favorite muffin for making croutons is Foods By George® English Muffins—look for them in the freezer of your health food store. Another good choice is French Bread—Glutino®. They make a par-baked loaf that is perfect for croutons.

Ingredients

3 GF English Muffins or 6 slices French bread

1/4 cup CF margarine, melted (or olive oil)

1 clove garlic, minced

Salt, pepper to taste

Preheat oven to 350°.

Cut muffins or bread into cubes and place in large bowl. In a large sauté pan, melt margarine (or heat oil). Add garlic and cook for 1 minute. Stir in bread and toss until well coated.

Place in a single layer on a greased cookie sheet. Bake until the cubes are dry on one side, then turn them with a spatula and toast the other side. Check often to prevent burning.

Hail Caesar Dressing

We love Caesar Salads, and often my husband makes them with grilled chicken meat or boiled shrimp and we call it a meal. Though many children do not like vegetables, Caesar Salad is often an exception. Add some grilled chicken strips for added protein.

Blend together:

3/4 cup GF mayonnaise

3 tablespoons white rice vinegar

2 tablespoons Soymage grated parmesan "cheese"

2 teaspoons Worcestershire sauce

1/2 teaspoon lemon juice

1/2 teaspoon ground dry mustard

1/4 teaspoon salt

1/4 teaspoon garlic powder

1/4 teaspoon onion powder

1/4 teaspoon ground black pepper

Pinch dried basil

Pinch dried oregano

1 "squirt" anchovy paste*

Combine all ingredients in a blender and blend until smooth.

*Available in most grocery stores

Ranch Salad Dressing or Dip

I often hear from parents who say that their children used to eat vegetables, but only if they were dipped in Ranch dressing. This is a pretty good facsimile of a true Ranch dressing. Ranch dressing usually contains a lot of sweetening in the form of sugar and corn syrup. If tolerated, you may want to add a teaspoon of one of these sweeteners. Although DariFree is my favorite milk substitute, the vanilla flavor does not work well for Ranch dressing! I recommend a soy based milk if tolerated, or coconut milk.

Ingredients

1 cup GF mayonnaise

1 cup milk substitute with 1 teaspoon lemon juice added

2 tablespoons onion powder

1/2 teaspoon dried parsley

1/4 teaspoon garlic powder

1/4 teaspoon black pepper

Salt to taste (start with 1/4 teaspoon)

1 teaspoon xanthan gum

Combine in blender.   Store in refrigerator.

Thousand Island Dressing & Dip

This was a mainstay in our household when I was growing up. Because it is a bit sweet, you may be able to persuade your kids to eat some salad or at the very least, to dip a carrot stick. If you've got some dill pickles in the fridge, a little of the "juice" is a great addition. In some parts of the country this is called Russian Dressing, but it's the same thing.

Ingredients

1 cup GF/CF mayonnaise

1/4 cup (or more, to taste) ketchup

2 tablespoons sweet pickle relish

1/4 teaspoon celery seed

1 teaspoon sugar (or substitute)

1 tablespoon dill pickle juice (optional)

Salt, pepper (to taste)

Combine all ingredients in a small bowl. Keep refrigerated.

Apple Pie Spice

Lots of muffin and quick bread recipes call for this simple spice. It is easy to make your own. Spices lose their kick after six months to a year, so don't make this or other spice blends in too large a batch.

Ingredients

4 parts cinnamon

2 parts nutmeg (freshly grated if possible)

1 part ground cardamom

Combine all ingredients and store in an airtight glass jar.

Japanese Ginger Dressing and Dip

Every Japanese restaurant I've ever been to uses a ginger-based dressing for their salad. Annie's Naturals® makes a very good version, but it is not gluten free. Fortunately it is easy to make at home.

Ingredients

1/2 cup minced onion

1/2 cup sunflower oil

1/3 cup rice vinegar

2 tablespoons water

2 tablespoons minced fresh ginger

2 tablespoons ketchup

4 teaspoons GF Worcestershire sauce

2 teaspoons sugar

2 teaspoons lemon juice

1/2 teaspoon minced garlic

1/2 teaspoon salt

1/4 teaspoon black pepper

Combine all ingredients in a blender. Blend on high speed for about 30 seconds or until all of the ginger is well pureed.

Seasoned Salt

Some kids hate spice, and others won't eat anything without it. Here is a tasty blend that will work well when roasting or broiling meat. It is also good on vegetables. Try sprinkling some on oven French fries.

Ingredients

2 tablespoons salt

1 teaspoon sugar

1/2 teaspoon imported paprika

1/4 teaspoon turmeric

1/4 teaspoon onion powder

1/4 teaspoon garlic powder

1/4 teaspoon potato starch

Combine all ingredients and mix well. Store tightly covered in a small jar.

Pumpkin Pie Spice

Here's another one that is called for in many recipes. I never trust spice blends to be free of additives, so I prefer to make my own.

Ingredients

4 parts cinnamon

2 parts ground ginger

1 part ground mace

1 part ground cloves

1 part nutmeg (freshly grated if possible)

Combine all ingredients and store in an airtight glass jar.

Taco Seasoning Mix

Lots of recipes call for taco seasoning, but you will be safer if you make it yourself from spices you know to be gluten free. Always check with manufacturers; spices often contain flour to prevent clumping. There are several brands that do not, but you should check occasionally to be sure.*

Ingredients

2 teaspoons onion powder

1 teaspoon chili powder

1/2 teaspoon crushed dried red pepper

1/4 teaspoon dried oregano

1 teaspoon salt

1/2 teaspoon tapioca starch

1/2 teaspoon garlic powder

1/2 teaspoon ground cumin

Mix all ingredients and store in an airtight container. This makes the equivalent of one envelope of taco seasoning.

*As of this writing, McCormick spices are gluten free. Always check with manufacturers however, and keep track of ingredient changes on a list such as the one kept at **www.gfcfdiet.com.**

Onion Soup Mix

There was a time when just about every recipe used a packet of Lipton's® Onion Soup mix. They now make one variety (Recipe Secrets) that is gluten free. It is filled, however, with the usual preservatives and additives that you may want to avoid. It is easy to make your own, and the mix is great for adding to casseroles and meat loaves. This recipe makes the equivalent of one packet.

Ingredients

1/4 cup dehydrated minced onion

2 tablespoons GF beef or vegetable bouillon

1/2 teaspoon onion powder

1/2 teaspoon salt

Combine all ingredients. Store in airtight jar.

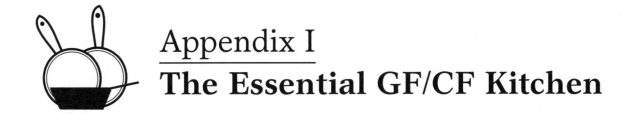

Appendix I
The Essential GF/CF Kitchen

Equipping a kitchen for the special dietary needs of autistic spectrum children is not terribly different from outfitting any kitchen. However, if you are not converting your kitchen to all-GF/CF, you will need to be very careful about cross-contamination. There are some ways to greatly reduce the chances of an "accident," and you will want to keep a few pieces of equipment for use with GF/CF ingredients only.

I love kitchen appliances and gadgets, and have always had many of them. The fact is that most are luxuries, however, and not necessary. The following is a list of the appliances I recommend or about which I am asked the most.

Highly Recommended Items

Stand Mixer   A good mixer is a necessity. If you do not have a stand mixer, be sure that you have a very strong hand mixer. A good stand mixer, like a KitchenAid® or Kenwood®, is expensive, but well worth the expense. I have had the same KitchenAid® for fifteen years! I use it nearly every day. I make GF breads in the mixer.

Food Processor   A food processor is another recommended appliance, although a very good blender will work, too. Nothing beats a food processor when it comes to shredding or grating, and many people use their food processor as I use my mixer. If you cannot have both a mixer and a food processor, my preference is for the mixer. Not everyone agrees. If you do not have a stand mixer, you will need a food processor.

Blender

Most people have a blender and it is worth the expense to have a good one. For years I coveted the VitaMix® blender, but I could not bring myself to spend the $400-plus to get one. I decided to look on eBay (online auction) and found a ten year old Vita-mix® for a very reasonable price. Because, like good mixers, they last "forever," I felt comfortable buying it used. I have not regretted it. It blends, it grinds, it mixes—you can even freeze "ice cream" or cook soup. I have not scratched the surface of what it can do, but it's been a great addition to my kitchen. You don't need a fancy blender, but you do need a good one with a strong motor. If you have a really good food processor, you can probably do without this.

Toaster Oven

I have always preferred a toaster to a toaster oven, mostly because a toaster takes up so much less room on the counter. If you are going to cook both GF and regular foods, however, a toaster oven is a much better choice. I have two toaster oven trays so that I never use Sam's tray for his brother's gluten breads or muffins. A toaster is also much harder to clean than a toaster oven, and even a few errant crumbs can be a problem. I strongly suggest a toaster oven, and if counter space is a problem try an "under the counter" model.

Wooden Spoons

Be sure you have a set that are used only for GF/CF cooking. These essential implements are nearly impossible to clean completely.   (Although you might be interested to know that I read a study that said that wood utensils retained fewer bacteria—after washing—than either metal or plastic. —ed).

Waffle Iron

Waffle irons are great, and I would not be without one. However, cleaning between all those little projections is difficult. I never feel that it is completely cleaned and for that reason, I make only GF waffles on my waffle iron. There are many excellent GF pancake/waffle mixes, and *Special Diets for Special Kids* included several scratch recipes. When we eat homemade waffles, we all eat GF ones. If you must make "regular" waffles and GF ones, I recommend you keep two separate irons. Note: there are excellent frozen GF waffles available, but they are expensive.

Cookie Sheets

I use only insulated cookie sheets. These are cookie sheets made of two layers of metal, separated by air. They greatly reduce the number of burned cookies! I really recommend these insulated sheets.

Silpat mats	I know that many would consider these rather expensive mats luxury items, but they are on my "must have" list! A silpat is a reusable, rubberized-silicone mat that makes any baking sheet nonstick. Cookies and buns lift right off and make scrubbing baking sheets a thing of the past. I recently discovered that my silpat mats are the perfect surface on which to roll out dough. This eliminates scraping bits of dough from my countertop and the whole piece of dough can be lifted easily—especially nice when rolling out a piecrust. These mats are expensive, but well worth it. Buy at least one—more if you can.
Pastry Blender	An old-fashioned pastry blender is probably buried in the bottom of your kitchen's junk drawer. It is a simple and inexpensive implement, just a wooden handle and four or five pieces of wire curved around it. It is indispensable, however, when trying to evenly blend margarine into a flour mixture. They are very inexpensive, so if you can't find one in your kitchen, be sure to purchase one at a kitchen supply store.

Not Essential, But Recommended

Coffee Grinder	No, I don't recommend you start giving your children coffee! A coffee grinder is a small but powerful grinder that also works for spices or grains (in very small batches of course). A coffee grinder is also useful for making powdered sugar (important if you are avoiding corn). If you also grind coffee beans, buy a second one that you use exclusively for non-coffee grinding jobs.

Deep Fryer   A deep fryer is a great appliance to have, though a deep pan will work for most frying jobs. Nuggets, fries and other fried foods taste great if truly "deep" fried. Do not pollute your oil with gluten filled breadings.

Pastry bags
& tubes   If you have never used a pastry bag fitted with a decorative tip (or tube), you probably believe it is hard to do. It isn't! Like anything else, using a pastry bag takes a little practice if you want the results to look really nice. Even if you'll never be a master cake decorator, these are very useful to have in the kitchen, and you can even buy an inexpensive set with disposable bags. Next time you have some leftover mashed potatoes, put them in the bag and practice!

Potato Ricer   For the ultimate fluffy, light mashed potatoes, for chunk (or smooth) applesauce, or for coarse (or fine) mashed root vegetables, try a potato ricer. It looks like a giant garlic press and is a very useful gadget to own.

Luxury Items—Nice if you Can Afford Them

Bread Machine

I am often asked whether or not a bread machine is necessary and my answer has changed. I used to believe that it was important to have a bread machine, but have come to believe that it is one of the more unnecessary appliances. Why? Because the point of a bread machine is to save the work of all that kneading, and GF breads do not require kneading. Kneading is done to develop the gluten in yeast breads—since GF breads have no gluten there is little point in kneading. Gluten free bread dough is more like cake batter and should be treated that way. In general, kneading will cause GF breads to be coarse textured, and is completely unnecessary. I have a bread machine, but use it only rarely.

Ice cream machine

There are many kinds of ice cream machines on the market, ranging in price from under $30 to several thousand! A luxury item to some, you will find it a wonderful addition to the kitchen if you want to make delicious, (corn-free) frozen desserts for your family. I again turned to an on-line auction when I wanted a new ice cream maker, and I love it. I recommend the type that has a frozen bowl onto which you fit a combination cover/motor/stirring mechanism. I keep the bowl in the freezer between uses, so I can make ice cream whenever the mood strikes. My family considers this machine one of my best purchases ever!

Rice Cooker	Many GF families have rice so frequently that a rice cooker seems like a good investment. If money and counter space are no problem, you will probably enjoy having this appliance. It is certainly not necessary however, and does belong on the luxury list. I have recently found that the microwave is an excellent way to cook rice, and allows me to cook, serve and store the rice all in the same casserole dish. A real plus in my opinion!
Pizzelles iron	This iron is used for making Pizzelles, a traditional egg-and-butter cookie flavored with anise, rum or vanilla (see recipe, page 212). When hot off the iron, these cookies can be formed into cones (for sorbet or non-dairy ice cream). I like to place the hot cookies over the back of a custard cup to cool into the shape of the cup. Then the kids eat their ice cream AND the cup, which they think is pretty funny. Authentic Foods® pancake mix makes a terrific pizelle cookie.

Doughnut pan

Making baked doughnuts is really simple when you have one of the new non-stick doughnut pans. Available for full size doughnuts or minis, this is a great item to have in the kitchen.

Hamburger Bun Pan

Chicago Metallic® manufactures and King Arthur Flour both sell a terrific pan for making your own hamburger buns. It is an 11 x 16-inch aluminized steel pan that makes six big 4-inch buns. It'll hold a typical 3-cup flour-dough recipe, and is a great boon for those of us who cannot simply pick up a package of buns at the store.

English Muffin Rings

These rings generally come in sets of four, and are very inexpensive. They are terrific for making many things that you want to keep round. And of course, you may want to try making your own English muffins.

Appendix II
The GF/CF Pantry

When you first start following a gluten and casein free diet, the grocery store suddenly becomes a much less friendly place, with hidden sources of gluten and casein lurking in the least likely places. Learning what foods and what ingredients to avoid takes time and patience, and possibly a good pair of reading glasses to see all those tiny lists printed on the sides of food packages.

I always try to remind people of all the foods that **can** be eaten before listing the ones that cannot. There is no reason to restrict fruits, vegetables, meat, fish or fowl. You may need to change the way some of these foods are prepared or the condiments served with them, but most fresh foods are fine. In general, the less preparation involved the more likely a food is "safe." Of course, these are not the foods our children generally choose, so shopping sometimes feels like a stroll through a minefield.

I am often asked for a list of brand name foods that contain no harmful proteins, but unfortunately this is not always a safe approach. Food manufacturers often change ingredients, so a food that was on an approved food list last month may not be safe anymore. You should always check a source such as **www.gfcfdiet.com**, which keeps up-to-date food lists and alerts visitors to status changes. You should also make a habit of calling food companies. All the big companies can tell you which of their foods are appropriate. Be aware, too, that a product may be GF if produced in the United States, but contain gluten if produced elsewhere (even though the food has the same name). For example, a recent inquiry to Lea & Perrins® turned up the information that American produced Lea

& Perrins® Worcestershire Sauce is gluten free; the same product, purchased in Canada, contains gluten!

What about cross-contamination? Many times food producers will not guarantee that a food is gluten or casein free, even though they do not add any gluten or casein containing products to the food. If they produce gluten or casein containing foods on the same equipment, there is always the possibility of cross-contamination. In most cases, equipment is carefully cleaned between runs and it is highly unlikely that the food will present a problem. In order to avoid litigation, however, the company will simply not guarantee the gluten-free status of the foods.

Are these foods safe? They probably are, in the vast majority of cases. You must make the decision yourself on whether to use such foods, however, and be on the lookout for any negative reactions to foods produced in these factories.

In my opinion, cross-contamination is more of a risk when eating in restaurants. Most restaurants fry potatoes in the same oil used for other (breaded) foods. Even if they do not use the same oil on a given day, the oils are often strained and combined at the end of the day. Such straining is not enough to prevent contamination. Fast food restaurants have strict rules about combining oils—but you must check with the managers to see that these rules are actually being followed. Accidental contamination can happen after cooking too; my son has found (breaded) onion rings in his Burger King® French fries.

Most books on gluten free cooking state that white (grain) vinegar must be avoided, as well as any product that has alcohol (e.g., vanilla extract). For years the debate has raged on in the celiac community—can you use "grain" vinegar or foods that contain it? Celiac societies insist that such foods are not safe, while food scientists insist that they are. It is understandable, of course, that people who become ill, sometimes violently, err on the side of caution. On the other hand, why ask these scientists for their opinions and then ignore their response?

I can only report what the experts have said. Dr. Don Kasarda, for example, is a respected U.S. grain chemist who has provided research-based information to celiac groups for many years. Asked repeatedly about vinegar, Dr. Kasarda's answer remains steadfast:

"Amino acids, peptides and proteins are of such low volatility compared to the high volatility of ethyl alcohol that they should not be found in the distilled alcohol. There is no scientific evidence for gluten peptides in alcohol or vinegar that I am aware of. I have never encountered a single chemist who thinks there are gluten peptides in distilled alcohol from wheat grain. I have not personally researched this matter because it is such an unlikely possibility and to prove the absence of gluten peptides that might be present in minute amounts is likely to be a major, costly undertaking and not at all easy. I realize that some celiac patients may have a disagreeable digestive response to white vinegar...but if it doesn't bother you don't worry about it. If it does bother you, don't ingest it. Malt vinegar is the only vinegar that I think might contain harmful peptides."

Do I recommend that you stop worrying about vinegar? What about alcohol-based flavorings like vanilla extract? I believe that these foods are safe, but this is a decision that you will have to make for yourself. If your child is one who shows a dramatic behavioral response to ingesting even a minute quantity of gluten, you should be able to determine quickly whether or not it is something to include in the diet.

A conservative approach would be to use cider vinegar when cooking and making foods such as salad dressings; use glycerin-based or powdered vanilla and other extracts; include foods that use vinegar (but are free of gluten) with caution. In other words, use your best judgment.

Another area of equivocation involves oats. Recent research is indicating that oats may be a safe food for gluten-intolerant people. In my opinion it is probably too early to declare oats safe for gluten intolerant individuals, but it may happen. For now it is best to avoid oats along with wheat, rye and barley products.

So, what to buy, cook and eat? This is a moving target of course, but there are foods that must be avoided and foods that are nearly always OK (unless there is a food allergy).

Gluten-Containing Ingredients

Wheat (including Spelt, triticale and Kamut)

Rye

Barley

Oats

Ingredients Which Often Contain Gluten*

Malt

Malt flavoring

MSG (Monosodium Glutamate)

Hydrolyzed Vegetable Protein

Rice Syrup (GF rice syrup is available and is so designated)

Natural flavorings

Artificial flavors

Artificial colors

Dextrin

Dextrose

Caramel Color

*These ingredients may or may not contain gluten. The only way to be sure is to call the food's manufacturer. Dextrin, for example, is usually corn-derived but could come from other sources. Caramel color produced in this country is almost always gluten free, but a food may have another source for its caramel. The caramel in Coca-Cola® is GF, for example, but other sources may not be safe. Always check. Many of these ingredients (e.g., Dextrin and dextrose) usually have a corn source, so if avoiding corn you must be doubly cautious.

Hidden Sources of Gluten

Frozen potatoes (often conveyer belts are dusted with flour to prevent sticking)

Bulk raisins (again, flour dusting is common)

Gravy

Tuna fish (generally GF but may contain casein)

Tomato paste

Prepackaged yeast (some yeasts are grown on wheat sources)

Confectioner's sugar (may contain flour and/or cornstarch)

Sirimi/imitation crabmeat

Flavorings

Commercially ground spices

Vitamins

Medications (both over the counter and prescription medications use fillers)

Candy

Chewing gum

Condiments

Envelope glue

Postage Stamps

Playdoh®

School glue

Tropical fish flake food

Dairy Products and Ingredients To Avoid

Cow's milk

Butter

Margarines (unless completely dairy-free)

Yogurt

Powdered milk

Cheese

Whey

Lactose

Casein

Caseinate

Sodium caseinate

Cottage Cheese

Ricotta Cheese

Anything that is derived from the milk of a bovine animal!

Nursing mothers: Yes, human milk contains casein, but it is a far smaller percentage of the milk protein than found in bovine milks. Mothers should continue to nurse their babies, but if they already have an autistic child, or if the nursing child is on the autistic spectrum, the mother should remove all dairy and gluten-containing products from her diet. These have been shown to pass through the breast milk. Work with a doctor or nutritionist to ensure that adequate calcium and other nutrients are eaten.

Foods and Ingredients To Have In Your Pantry

There are many grains and flours that are safe for you to use, and these are listed below. Often these grains and flours are available only through mail order or from health food stores. If your health food store carries these in bulk bins, you will save money— but you may want to be wary of bulk buying—customers are often careless and use the same scoops in more than one bin! Cross-contamination is a real likelihood in these situations. Mail order suppliers are probably a safer choice for specialty grains and flours (see Appendix III). **Please note: any brand names mentioned in this chapter are gluten and casein free as of this writing. Always read labels and check with manufacturers.**

Safe Grains and Alternative Flours Made From Them

Brown rice & flour

White rice & flour

Sweet rice flour (sometimes called glutinous)

Potato starch

Potato flour

Tapioca Flour (often called tapioca starch or tapioca starch flour)

Cornstarch (though many are sensitive to corn)

Arrowroot Starch (use in place of cornstarch if corn-sensitive)

Soy flour (many are sensitive to soy)

Chickpeas (also called garbanzos)

Chickpea flour (also called besan)

Garfava flour (combination of Chickpeas and Fava Beans)

Sorghum flour (also called Jowar)*

Peas and pea flours*

Lentils (also called pulses)*

Amaranth

Buckwheat (kasha)

Buckwheat flour

Millet

Rice Polish

Teff

Wild rice

Quinoa

Seeds and nuts (toasted or dry roasted)

*If you can find an Indian or Indo-Pak grocery store, you will find these and hundreds of different lentils and flours available to you, often at prices far less than those of health food stores. Chinese markets are another good source of rice products.

Using GF Flours

When cooking or baking without wheat, it is important to use a combination of flours. While a few recipes call for only one type of flour (usually white rice), the vast majority will work better if you use a combination of flours. By combining flours, you reduce the crumbly-ness of a food and enhance the finished product. The addition of bean flours adds protein, flavor and moistness to GF baked goods.

Bette Hagman (the original Gluten-Free Gourmet) has created wonderful flour combinations that work in a variety of recipes. Her combinations are so useful that many of the mail order companies now sell them, pre-mixed. Initially I assumed that mixing the flours myself would save money, but in fact, there is little difference and I usually buy the flours pre-mixed and in large quantities. It is useful to have the formulas, however, because you may not have the flour mixture you want at a given time. If you are rotating foods, it is important to have a few different flour combinations so that you can, for example, have a flour to use on a rice-free day.

In the recipes in this book, I have specified only "GF Flour blend." My favorite flours are Hagman's Featherlight flour, Hagman's Four Flour Bean Mix and Gift of Nature® blend. Sometimes, I use sorghum flour alone—this flour is probably the closest to wheat flour available to us. More often, I use sorghum for $1/2$ to $3/4$ of the flour and a flour mix for the rest. Bob's Red Mill® makes "white" sorghum that is excellent for GF baking. To get the texture and taste your family prefers, you may want to experiment.

When I bake, I use one teaspoon xanthan or guar gum for each cup of flour. If you make your own flour blends, it is a time-saver to add the gum to the flour mixture. Be sure to stir together all ingredients until evenly blended. All the following flour mixtures can be purchased premixed (see Appendix III.)

A Note about guar gum: In her first book, *The Gluten Free Gourmet,* Bette Hagman mentions that guar gum may have a laxative effect. For this reason most people avoid using it in favor of (the far more expensive) xanthan gum. The fact is, for the vast majority of people guar gum causes no discernible problem. Further, many children on the autistic spectrum are actually constipated (see comment on page 45) and therefore any possible laxative effect may really be beneficial. Because guar gum is generally far cheaper than xanthan gum, it is certainly reasonable to try it. It can be used in place of guar gum in any recipe in this book, exchanged measure for measure.

Hagman's Basic GF Flour Mix

This is Hagmans' original flour mix. It is a bit grainy but is a good basic flour replacer.

2 parts rice flour (white or brown)

1 part potato starch

1 part tapioca flour

Hagman's Four Flour Bean Mix

*Hagman created this mixture for her book, **The Gluten-Free Gourmet Bakes Bread**. This is a fantastic flour, and one I use all the time. According to Hagman, "this flour may revolutionize gluten-free baking." She is right—it can be used in a cup-for-cup exchange of wheat flour for most recipes. It's terrific. If you need to avoid corn, you will have to make this yourself substituting arrowroot for the cornstarch.*

1 part garfava bean flour (available from Authentic Foods®)

1 part sorghum flour

1 part cornstarch (use arrowroot if corn intolerant)

1 part tapioca flour

Hagman's Featherlight Rice Flour Mix

This is a wonderfully versatile flour mix. I buy it in five pound bags from Miss Roben's and use it often. It is lighter than the basic rice mix. Because it has no beans, the protein content is lower than the Four Flour Bean Mix. It is harder to use this flour when adapting wheat recipes, but I often use this in combination with bean flours. Because it is a lighter flour, I tend to use it for cakes rather than breads. If avoiding corn, make your own using arrowroot starch.

I part rice flour

I part tapioca flour

I part cornstarch

Potato flour (not potato starch)—one teaspoon per cup of flour blend

Other Gluten-Free Ingredients To Have on Hand*

Bean thread (noodles)

Bouillon—use when broth is not available.

GF bread or cracker crumbs—great for breading nuggets or fish sticks.

GF bread (there are many brands available, vacuum sealed or frozen)

Breakfast cereal—there are now many varieties available. Use for breakfast or for baking.

Broth, chicken and beef—use for low fat sautéing, and adding flavor to casseroles.

Coconut, unsweetened—use in place of sweetened coconut. Adds bulk when baking with sugar substitutes.

Coconut butter—non-dairy fat for baking or frying. Has very high smoke point.

Coconut milk, regular and light—great as milk substitute in casseroles and baked goods.

"Cream" soups—useful for sauces; look for Imagine® brand soups.

Guar gum—can be used instead of xanthan gum.

Kudzu—a great thickener to use when making CF puddings. Often puddings do not thicken properly when made without real milk. Kudzu will help pudding "set."

Mashed potato flakes (sulfite free)—excellent filler for soups and casseroles. Useful in breading recipes.

Nutriflax Powder—adds fiber and essential fatty acids to baked goods.

Pasta—available in various shapes made from rice, corn, quinoa and blends.

Sunflower seeds—adds protein and crunch to cereals and baked goods.

Tofu (if soy is tolerated—excellent source of protein in soups and casseroles). Versatile.

(Frozen) waffles—far more expensive than homemade, but great for those hurried mornings. There are a few GF brands available (e.g. Van's and Waffle House).

Xantham gum—use for all gluten free baking.

*See Appendix VI for any terms you do not know.

Appendix III
Finding a Good GF Bread*

*F*inding a bread that kids will eat may be the single hardest part of following a GF/CF diet. It is impossible to name **the** best bread, recipe or mix, since different people look for different qualities in the bread they enjoy. We decided it made sense to ask **ANDI News** readers what breads they recommend, and what they like and dislike about their choices. What follows was written using the comments of over 100 parents following the GF diet.

As expected, store-bought breads were rated best for convenience, but worst for price, taste and texture. Most require toasting to be palatable. Mixes are also expensive, but are very popular due to convenience and the great taste of a loaf right out of the oven. Most find that GF/CF breads turn out best when made at home.

A sampling of positive and negative comments follows.

Favorite Store-Bought Breads

Food For Life® White Rice Bread

"In addition to gluten and casein, it is free of eggs, soy, corn, nuts. It tastes good, doesn't fall apart, and makes good sandwiches. We find the texture and taste to be the closest to regular bread. All of our kids like it when it is toasted. Sometimes it's too mushy when it defrosts. It's thinly cut so it's great for sandwiches but the frozen slices can stick together and be hard to pull apart. Its texture has improved recently."

*This appendix was excerpted from an article that originally appeared in *The ANDI News,* 2001, Vol. 4 (2).

Food for Life® Brown Rice Bread

"Great texture, looks like whole wheat, very moist, great flavor, fruit juice sweetened. It doesn't contain arrowroot or nuts. Toasted, it has a good flavor and consistency, but it can be difficult to separate the frozen slices." I have to partially defrost the loaf, then separate the slices and refreeze, with the slices stacked differently. It is close enough in color to wheat bread to pass my son's test. It works well ground up as breadcrumbs."

Ener-G Foods® Tapioca Bread

"It is white and it looks like regular bread, but I dislike the texture and the flavor. My kids will eat it with honey or fruit spread, but they won't eat it plain. It doesn't 'soak up' well for French toast, but it's the only bread our son likes. Good for bread crumbs. My son likes this bread better than other store brands ... though I think it tastes like a sponge."

Other Favorites

Food for Life® Pecan and Rice Bread

"The pieces are too small and the bread is a little dense for me, but this is a good substitute when I am too busy to bake. The flavor is excellent, and it contains no corn products."

Ener-G Foods® Brown Rice Yeast-Free Loaf

"The only commercially available bread in our area without yeast. It has a gummy texture, but I keep some in the freezer in case we run out of homemade bread. It looks like 'regular' white bread, is softer than many brands, and I like that it is yeast free. Must be toasted."

Noah's Bread and variations

"It's soft, holds it's shape, and is versatile. You can add all kinds of ingredients to make it different. Most important, it's very easy and has come out great for me." "It is yeast-free and the air holes caused by the sparkling water create a taste and effect similar to air bagels. I *love* this bread because it is soft and chewy and passes as real bread. I make it with bean flours and even my son likes it!" [Note: Miss Roben's is now selling a Noah's Bread mix.]

Marci's Soft White Bread from *Special Diets for Special Kids* and *Unraveling the Mystery of Autism and PDD*

"The best bread we have made for my daughter and she eats it like regular bread. It is soft, freezes great and microwaves great too. It is easy to make, and has a really smooth texture. Makes great rolls. Good taste and texture when it comes out. Not always successful; loaves can collapse. It smells great when it's baking, has wonderful flavor and makes great toast. It is my son's favorite! Two small loaves work better than one large one."

Basic Featherlight Rice Bread from *The Gluten-free Gourmet Bakes Bread*

"Very tasty and has a great texture. It doesn't crumble and stays nice for a week. Don't over bake."

Bette Hagman's Yeast-free Basic Almond Bread (6%) from *The Gluten-free Gourmet Bakes Bread*

"Uses 4 flour bean mix. It is consistently springy, tasty and nutritious. It is a forgiving recipe that allows changes such as reducing the sugar, adding rice polish or flax meal, and using eggs instead of egg substitutes. Keeps well."

Yeast-free White Bread from *Special Diets for Special Kids*

"My son likes it, and it's easy to prepare but it hardens quickly. I have to make small amounts fresh almost daily."

Sorghum Bread from *The Gluten-Free Gourmet Bakes Bread*

"Very close to wheat bread. It works best when made by hand, and is relatively low in protein and fiber."

French Bread from *The Gluten Free Gourmet Bakes Bread*

"Good flavor and texture similar to real French bread, but a little heavier. Leftovers do not keep very well."

Yeast Free Sandwich Bread from *Special Diet Solutions*

"A good sandwiches loaf—soft and pleasant tasting. Slightly dense and heavy texture due to lack of yeast but despite this is the best tasting yeast-free bread I have made."

Favorite Mixes

Miss Roben's ANDI Wunderbread

"Easy, and it comes out great every time.   Makes great rolls. You can make bagels (leave out yeast and vinegar and pipe it onto a cookie sheet or donut pan). Delicious."

Authentic Foods® Cinnamon Raisin Bread

"My son and I both like the mix. I have found bread making to be very challenging."

Miss Roben's White Sandwich Bread Mix

"I dumped it in the bread machine. It made the best loaf and tasted good, too. I like that it can be made without yeast."

Gluten Free Pantry's Favorite Sandwich Bread

"I add two teaspoons of a Dough Enhancer, also ordered from the Gluten Free Pantry to increase the shelf life of the loaf of bread. I divide it into three parts and freeze two of them."

My son Sam likes *Food For Life*® **Rice Pecan** and the new *Ener-G Foods*® **Seattle Brown Bread.** Seattle Brown bread is as close as I have tasted to "honey wheat." Like all Ener-g breads, it really LOOKS good. It holds together well and while it makes good toast you don't *have* to toast it. It contains corn so not everyone will be able to use it. I also really like **Kinnikinnick** Foods breads and rolls, and some can usually be found in my freezer.

ANDI Wunderbread, adapted by Miss Robens from **Special Diets,** has great flavor and a crunchy crust (which we like). I do not think it works well as a large bread but it makes terrific rolls. I recently discovered White Bread mix from **Authentic Foods.** It takes a little more work than most mixes but it has a terrific texture, rises high and tastes great.

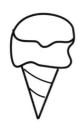

Appendix IV
Ice Cream Fundamentals

by Diane Hartman

If you ask anyone on a dairy free diet what they miss most, the answer will nearly always be ice cream! (I've yet to hear anyone moan about missing cottage cheese!) I am a firm believer in finding good tasting, satisfying substitutions for beloved foods, because unless you do, your efforts are likely doomed to failure. If your children feel deprived, they will find a way to get what they want.

Fortunately, there are now some wonderful dairy-free sorbets available. And because everyone is watching their fat intake, the major ice cream makers have gotten into the sorbet business. Hagen-Dasz, Ben & Jerry's and many other brands are now easily found in any grocery store freezer. These are delicious, but for corn or soy intolerant children, they are usually off limits.

Even if you can eat corn products, there is something particularly wonderful about homemade ice creams and sorbets. Making dairy and gluten free ice cream is not really all that difficult, and it is gratifying to do because you can duplicate family favorites. In order to be successful, however, it is important to understand the function of various ingredients.

*Diane Hartman understands just what is necessary to make a good dairy free ice cream, and has explained it very clearly. This information was written for her own cookbook, **The Food Allergy Kitchen Children's Cookbook**. Diane has generously agreed to let me include this information here, and I know you will find it useful. Diane's book should be available during the 2002 calendar year, so keep your eyes open for it.*

Ingredient Functions in Dairy-Free Ice Cream

Liquids

Liquids are a required component in the formation of ice crystals. Ice crystals are a necessary element in the production of a solid dessert. It is important to remember that the water content of various liquids differs. The higher the water content of a liquid, the more significant the volume of ice crystal formation.

Sweeteners/Sugars

The intensity of sweetness in a frozen dessert is decreased as the temperature is reduced. Therefore, the liquid ice cream mixture may have an excessively sweet flavor but in the frozen stage may have a well-balanced sweet flavor.

Fat

Adding fat (oils, melted shortening, etc.) to a frozen dessert will aide in the production of a smooth texture. Coconut oil and canola oil are two good choices when selecting products to compose the fat content of a dairy free frozen dessert. Avoid using strongly flavored oils such as olive or safflower when making ice cream. The flavor of the fat used should be mild and not noticeable in the finished dessert.

Stabilizers/Emulsifiers

Gelatin, agar, guar gum, xanthan gum, etc., act as stabilizers and emulsifiers when incorporated into frozen desserts. These ingredients absorb and bind water. The absorption of the liquid reduces the crystal size, thus producing a smoother texture. However, excessive use of these items will result in a gummy and undesirable product.

Air

Introducing air via churning is a crucial factor in producing well-textured ice cream. The absence of air will result in a dense, coarse and grainy product. Air is most readily incorporated into the dessert mixture as it approaches the crystallization stage.

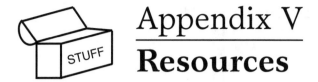

Appendix V
Resources

Vitamins and Supplements

http://www.kirkmanlabs.com:

Source for SupraNuThera vitamin-mineral complex and many other supplements
for autistic spectrum individuals, including EnzymeAid.

http://www.klaire.com:

Makers of SerenAide, a digestive enzyme.

Online Information and Support

Autism Network for Dietary Intervention: *http://www.AutismNDI.com*

The website I run with ANDI partner Karyn Seroussi. Contains helpful information and links as well as a Parent Support list sorted geographically (find some help
in YOUR neighborhood!).

GF/CF Kids: *http://www.gfcfdiet.com*

Good information AND a list of brand-name products!

The Feingold Association: *http://www.feingold.org*

Information on diet for ADHD, autism etc.

Allergy Induced Autism: *http://www.kessick.demon.co.uk/aia.htm*

It's the ANDI of the UK

Autism Research Unit (Paul Shattock's Group): *http://osiris.sunderland.ac.uk/autism/*

The Good News Foundation: *http://www.gnd.org/autism/autism.htm*

http://www.enabling.org/ia/celiac

The Living Sensibly Foundation: *http://www.livingsensibly.org/yourlife.asp*

The folks behind Vance's DariFree have put together this non-profit organization dedicated to improving health through diet

Sources of GF/CF Foods and Ingredients

http://www.vancesfoods.com:

For DariFree and related products

http://www.missroben.com:

My favorite mail order—The place to go for all your needs!

http://www.glutenfree.com:

One of the first and best sources for ingredients, mixes etc.

http://www.glutensolutions.com:

Another one-stop shopping experience.

http://www.glutenfree.com:

Check it out—lots of products.

http://www.authenticfoods.com:

Originators of Garfava flours and related products.

http://www.kinnikinnick.com:

Wonderful mixes, the best GF/CF donuts and by far the best GF pancake mix available today (in my opinion).

http://www.glutino.com:

Need pretzels? Great breadcrumbs? Incredible pasta? Look no further.

http://www.dietaryshoppe.com:

Lots of unusual products. Be sure to check it out.

http://www.giftsofnature.net:

Their basic flour blend is one of my all time favorites.

Information about Vaccines and Autism

These websites contain general information about vaccine safety and the possible connection to autism. Please check them out and do research before making any decisions about the vaccination schedule you choose for your children. Discuss this with your child's doctor, but make decisions based on knowledge, not medical dogma. Inform yourself about this very important topic.

http://tlredwood.home.mindspring.com/"

http://www.gti.net/truegrit/"

http://www.909shot.com

Books and Cookbooks

The Candida Control Cookbook, by Gail Burton (1993.) Published by Aslan Publishing. If you must avoid yeast, this is an excellent book.

Celiac Sprue: A Guide Through the Medicine Cabinet. Want to know if your child's medication contains gluten or milk products? Look no further! This book contains some basic information about gluten intolerance, and lists of mediations that are known to be free of gluten or gluten and milk products. To order, visit *http://www.stokesrx.com.* *Feast Without Yeast: 4 Stages Better Health: A Complete Guide To Implementing Yeast Free, Wheat (Gluten) Free and Dairy (Casein) Free Living* by Bruce Semon, MD and Lori Kornblum (1999) Wisconsin Inst. of Nutrition.

The Food Allergy Kitchen Children's Cookbook by Diane Hartman. To be published later this year.

The Gluten-Free Gourmet by Betty Hagman, (1991) Published by Henry Holt (paper)

The Gluten-Free Gourmet Bakes Bread : More Than 200 Wheat Free Recipes, by Bette Hagman (1999). Published by Henry Holt (hardcover)

The Gluten-Free Gourmet Cooks Fast and Healthy: Wheat-Free and Gluten-Free With No Fuss and Less Fat, by Bette Hagman, (1996) Published by Henry Holt (paper)

More from the Gluten-Free Gourmet : Delicious Dining Without Wheat, by Bette Hagman, (1994) Published by Henry Holt (paper)

Special Diet Celebrations: No Wheat, Gluten, Dairy, or Eggs by Carol Fenster, Ph.D. (1999) Published by The Savory Palate (paperback)

Special Diets for Special Kids, by Lisa S. Lewis, Ph.D. (1998). Published by Future Horizons, Inc., 721 W. Abram Street, Arlington, TX 76013. This is my first book. It has all the theory, history, and explanations for gluten free/casein free diets, and goes into more detail about sensitivity tests, symptoms, etc. It also contains 150 recipes. You can order it from Future Horizons (cost is $ 29.95). Their number is 800-489-0727, or fax your order with credit card information to 817-277-2270. Their website is **www.futurehorizons-autism.com.** They also publish a bi-monthly magazine, *The Autism-Asperger's Digest.* To subscribe ($44.95 per year) call the number above.

Special Diet Solutions: Healthy Cooking Without Wheat, Gluten, Dairy, Eggs, Yeast or Refined Sugar, by Carol Fenster Ph.D., (1997) Published by the Savory Palate (paper)

Unravelling the Mystery of Autism and Pervasive Developmental Disorder, by Karyn Seroussi (2000). Published by Simon & Schuster: NY.

Wheat-Free Recipes & Menus: Delicious Dining Without Wheat or Gluten, by Carol Fenster, Ph.D. Published by the Savory Palate. (paper)

ANDI
Autism Network for Dietary Intervention
P.O. Box 335
Pennington, NJ 08534-0335
Fax: 609-737-8453
Email: AutismNDI@aol.com
www.AutismNDI.com

The *ANDI News* is a quarterly, eight-page newsletter with articles by parents and professionals regarding their experiences with the diet. It includes the best gluten and casein-free recipes for picky, bread-loving children, kitchen tips, conference and research advisories, and mail-order for hard-to-find books and tapes.

Established in 1998 by authors Lisa Lewis (**Special Diets for Special Kids**), and Karyn *Seroussi (Unraveling the Mystery of Autism and PDD),* ANDI networks and supports families around the world who are beginning and maintaining a gluten & dairy-free diet for the treatment of autism.

For sample articles and lots of great info, visit *www.AutismNDI.com.*
Mail check or money order to: ANDI, PO Box 335, Pennington, NJ 08534-0335, USA.

Name _____

Address _____

City, State, Zip _____ , _____ _____

Phone (   ) _____ _____ Email "mail to: _____@_____.___ " _____@_____.___

Please enclose $24 for four issues of the 2001 calendar-year-based *ANDI News. International subscribers & Canadians please enclose $28 payable in U.S. dollars.*

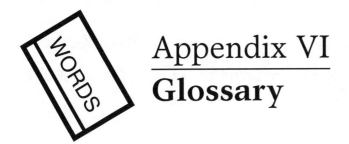

Appendix VI
Glossary

Agar A clear, flavorless sea vegetable. It is freeze-dried, sold in sticks, flakes or powder, and used like gelatin.

Amaranth Seeds that can be used as cereal, or ground into flour.

Arrowroot Starchy flour made from a tropical tuber. Can be substituted cup for cup for cornstarch.

Bean thread noodles Also called cellophane noodles. These translucent threads are made from the starch of green mung beans. Sold dried, they must be soaked briefly in hot water before using. They can also be deep-fried.

Brown Rice Syrup A thick, sweet syrup made from rice. Not all are GF. Read labels.

Casein One of the milk proteins. Must be avoided.

Coconut butter Refined from coconuts, this fat substitute works well in place of shortening. Very high smoke point, so it is excellent for frying.

Egg Replace   The brand name for a powdered combination of starches and leavening agents that bind cooked and baked foods in place of eggs.

Enterocolitis   Inflammations of both the small intestine and the colon.

Enteropathy   Disease of the intestines.

Eosinophilic Proctocolitis   Inflammation of the rectum and colon, characterized by infiltration of eosins into the tissues. Eosins are dyes used as stains in biology and pharmaceuticals.

Flax seeds   Tiny, oval-shaped brown seeds, also called linseeds. They are rich in omega-3 fatty acids. Very high in fiber. Can use a slurry of ground flaxseeds and water as an egg replacer in baked goods.

Gluten   A protein found in wheat, barley, rye and oats.

Guar gum   A vegetable gum that can be used as a binder in GF baking. Substitutes for the stretchiness of the gluten protein when baking bread with GF flours.

Histology   The study of cells and tissue at the microscopic level.

Hypoalbuminemia   Lack of albumen in the blood.   (Albumen is a protein and nutrient-carrying component of blood plasma.)

Kudzu   A white starchy powder made from the root of the kudzu plant. It is useful as a thickener for soups, sauces and puddings.

Millet   A tiny, round, golden, gluten-free grain. Is light and fluffy when cooked.

Miso   A salty paste made from cooked, aged soybeans and sometimes from other grains. Be sure to find miso that is gluten free. Avoid on yeast-free diet.

Poha   A staple of Indian cuisine, poha is another word for beaten rice. Poha is a flake that comes in thick and thin varieties. Thin poha makes a good substitute for oatmeal.

Polenta   A cornmeal mush that is a staple in Northern Italy. It is eaten hot like porridge or cooled and cut into squares that are sometimes grilled and served with marinara sauce.

Proctitis   Inflammation of the rectum.

Rice Paper Wrapper   Edible, translucent paper made from hot water and the pith of a tropical shrub. Sometimes rice flour is used.

Quinoa   A round, tan grain with a mild taste. High in protein.

Tahini   A thick smooth paste made of ground sesame seeds. Use in place of nut butters if nuts are not tolerated.

Tapioca   A starch extracted from the root of the cassava plant. Available in granules, flakes and "pearls". The flour is used in GF breads and for cooked puddings.

Tofu   White bean curd made from cooked soybeans. High in protein, it comes in soft, firm and extra firm styles. Can also be purchased in fat reduced varieties. Takes on the flavors of whatever foods it is cooked with.

Villus   (Plural: villi); A bacterium that lives in the human digestive system.

Xanthan gum   An emulsifier and stabilizer, this gum is made from fermented corn sugar. Most corn intolerant people can eat this without a problem. Substitutes for the stretchiness of the gluten protein when baking bread with GF flours.

Index